Quality Management for Health Care Delivery and Administration

About the Book

Healthcare administration relating to leadership, management, and administration of public health systems, health care systems, hospitals, and hospital networks. Health care administrators are considered health care professionals. Hospital administrators are individuals or groups of people who act as the central point of control within hospitals. These individuals may be previous or current clinicians, or individuals with other backgrounds. There are two types of administrators, generalists and specialists. Generalists are individuals who are responsible for managing or helping to manage an entire facility. Specialists are individuals who are responsible for the efficient operations of a specific department such as policy analysis, finance, accounting, budgeting, human resources, or marketing. Whether better administrators come from within or outside of the health profession is a matter of current debate.

About the Author

Dr. Ved Prakash, born on 1978, M.A, M.Phil, Political Science from J.N. University, Qualified the UGC NET is at presently Assistant Professor at K.R.Mahavidyalaya Chenari, Bihar, Under B.R.A. University. He is joined the college in 2007.He has specialisation in South Asia. He has attended four national and one International Level seminars and presented research papers.

Quality Management for Health Care Delivery and Administration

Dr. Ved Prakash

AMIGA PRESS INC.
DELHI (INDIA)

AMIGA PRESS INC.
H.O.: 28-A, Indra Park,
Chander Nagar, Delhi-110051 (India)
Tel.: 011-22504028, +91-98736-57000
E-mail: amigapress@gmail.com
amigaeditorial@gmail.com
amigapub@gmail.com
info@amigapress.co.in
Website : www.amigapress.co.in

This edition is published by Amiga Press Inc.

ISBN: 978-93-87295-28-5

First Published 2019

Printed and bound by Replika Press Pvt. Ltd.

Preface

Healthcare administration is the field relating to leadership, management, and administration of public health systems, health care systems, hospitals, and hospital networks. Health care administrators are considered health care professionals. Hospital administrators are individuals or groups of people who act as the central point of control within hospitals. These individuals may be previous or current clinicians, or individuals with other backgrounds. There are two types of administrators, generalists and specialists. Generalists are individuals who are responsible for managing or helping to manage an entire facility. Specialists are individuals who are responsible for the efficient operations of a specific department such as policy analysis, finance, accounting, budgeting, human resources, or marketing. Whether better administrators come from within or outside of the health profession is a matter of current debate.

Early hospital administrators were called patient directors or superintendents. At the time, many were nurses who had taken on administrative responsibilities. Over half of the members of the American Hospital Association were graduate nurses in 1916. Other superintendents were medical doctors, laymen and members of the clergy. In the United States, the first degree granting program in the United States was established at Marquette University in Milwaukee, Wisconsin. By 1927, the first two students received their degrees.

The original idea is credited to Father Moulinier, associated with the Catholic Hospital Association. The first modern health systems management program was established in 1934 at the University of Chicago. At the time, programs were completed in two years – one year of formal graduate study and one year of practicing internship. In 1958, the Sloan program at Cornell University began offering a special program requiring two years of formal study, which remains the dominant structure in the United States and Canada today. Health systems management has been described as a "hidden" health profession because of the relatively low-profile role managers take in health systems, in comparison to direct-care professions such as nursing and medicine. However the visibility of the management profession within healthcare has been rising in recent years, due largely to the widespread problems developed countries are having in balancing cost, access, and quality in their hospitals and health systems.

–Author

Contents

Chapter - 1

Introduction

Health care (or health care) is the diagnosis, treatment, and prevention of disease, illness, injury, and other physical and mental impairments in humans. Health care is delivered by practitioners in allied health, dentistry, midwifery- obstetrics, medicine, nursing, optometry, pharmacy and other care providers. It refers to the work done in providing primary care, secondary care, and tertiary care, as well as in public health.

Access to health care varies across countries, groups and individuals, largely influenced by social and economic conditions as well as the health policies in place. Countries and jurisdictions have different policies and plans in relation to the personal and population-based health care goals within their societies. Health care systems are organizations established to meet the health needs of target populations. Their exact configuration varies from country to country. In some countries and jurisdictions, health care planning is distributed among market participants, whereas in others planning is made more centrally among governments or other coordinating bodies. In all cases, according to the World Health Organization (WHO), a well-functioning health care system requires a robust financing mechanism; a well-trained and adequately-paid workforce; reliable information on which to base decisions and policies; and well maintained facilities and logistics to deliver quality medicines and technologies.

Health care can contribute to a significant part of a country's economy. In 2011, the health care industry consumed an average of 9.3 percent of the GDP orUS$ 3,322 (PPP-adjusted) per capita across the 34 members of OECD countries. The USA (17.7%, or US$ PPP 8,508), the Netherlands (11.9%, 5,099), France (11.6%, 4,118), Germany (11.3%, 4,495), Canada (11.2%, 5669), and Switzerland (11%, 5,634) were the top spenders, however life expectancy in total population at birth was highest in Switzerland (82.8 years), Japan and Italy (82.7), Spain and Iceland (82.4), France (82.2) and Australia (82.0), while OECD's average exceeds 80 years for the first time ever in 2011: 80.1 years, a gain of 10 years since 1970. The USA (78.7 years) ranges only on place 26 among the 34 OECD member countries, but has the highest costs by far. All OECD countries have achieved universal (or almost universal) health coverage, except Mexico and the USA.

Health care is conventionally regarded as an important determinant in promoting the general health and well-being of people around the world. An example of this is the worldwide eradication of smallpox in 1980—declared by the WHO as the first disease in human history to be completely eliminated by deliberate health care interventions.

DELIVERY OF MODERN HEALTH CARE

The delivery of modern health care depends on groups of trained professionals and paraprofessionalscoming together as interdisciplinary teams. This includes professionals in medicine, nursing, dentistry, midwifery- obstetrics and allied health, plus many others such as public health practitioners, community health workers and assistive personnel, who systematically provide personal and population-based preventive, curative and rehabilitative care services.While the definitions of the various types of health care vary depending on the different cultural, political, organizational and disciplinary perspectives, there appears to be some consensus that primary care constitutes the first element of a continuing health care process, that may also include the provision of secondary and tertiary levels of care. Health care can be defined as either public or private.

PRIMARY CARE

Primary care refers to the work of health care professionals who act as a first point of consultation for all patients within the health care system. Such a professional would usually be a primary care physician, such as a general practitioner or family physician, or a non-physician primary care provider, such as a physician assistant or nurse practitioner. Depending on the locality, health system organization, and sometimes at the patient's discretion, they may see another health care professional first, such as a pharmacist, a nurse (such as in the United Kingdom), a clinical officer (such as in parts of Africa), or an Ayurvedic or other traditional medicine professional (such as in parts of Asia). Depending on the nature of the health condition, patients may then be referred for secondary or tertiary care.

Primary care is often used as the term for the health care services which play a role in the local community. It can be provided in different settings, such as Urgent care centres which provide services to patients same day with appointment or walk-in bases.Primary care involves the widest scope of health care, including all ages of patients, patients of all socioeconomic and geographic origins, patients seeking to maintain optimal health, and patients with all manner of acute and chronic physical, mental and social health issues, including multiple chronic diseases. Consequently, a primary care practitioner must possess a wide breadth of knowledge in many areas. Continuity is a key characteristic of primary care, as patients usually prefer to consult the same practitioner for routine check-ups and preventive care, health education, and every time they require an initial consultation about a new health problem. The International Classification of Primary Care (ICPC) is a standardized tool for understanding and analyzing information on interventions in primary care by the reason for the patient visit.

Common chronic illnesses usually treated in primary care may include, for example: hypertension, diabetes, asthma, COPD, depression and anxiety, back pain, arthritis or thyroid dysfunction. Primary care also includes many basic maternal and child health care services, such as family planning services and vaccinations. In the United States, the 2013 National Health Interview Survey found that skin disorders (42.7%), osteoarthritis and joint disorders (33.6%), back problems (23.9%), disorders of lipid metabolism (22.4%), and upper respiratory tract disease (22.1%, excluding asthma) were the most common reasons for accessing a physician. In context of global population aging, with increasing numbers of older adults at greater risk of chronic non- communicable diseases, rapidly increasing demand for primary care services is expected around the world, in both developed and developing countries. The World Health Organization attributes the provision of essential primary care as an integral component of an inclusive primary health care strategy.

PHC AND POPULATION AGING

Given global demographic trends, with the numbers of people age 60 and over expected to double by 2025, PHC approaches have taken into account the need for countries to address the consequences of population ageing. In particular, in the future the majority of older people will be living in developing countries that are often the least prepared to confront the challenges of rapidly ageing societies, including high risk of having at least one chronic non- communicable disease, such as diabetes and osteoporosis. According to WHO, dealing with this increasing burden requires health promotion and disease prevention intervention at community level as well as disease management strategies within health care systems.

PHC AND MENTAL HEALTH

Some jurisdictions apply PHC principles in planning and managing their health care services for the detection, diagnosis and treatment of common mental health conditions at local clinics, and organizing the referral of more complicated mental health problems to more appropriate levels of mental health care.

SECONDARY CARE

Secondary care is the health care services provided by medical specialists and other health professionals who generally do not have first contact with patients, for example, cardiologists, urologists and dermatologists. It includes acute care: necessary treatment for a short period of time for a brief but serious illness, injury or other health condition, such as in a hospital emergency department. It also includes skilled attendance during childbirth, intensive care, and medical imaging services. The "secondary care" is sometimes used synonymously with "hospital care". However many secondary care providers do not necessarily work in hospitals, such as psychiatrists, clinical psychologists, occupational therapists or physiotherapists, and some primary care services are delivered within hospitals. Depending on the organization and policies of the national health system, patients may be required to see a primary care provider for a referral before they can access secondary care.

For example in the United States, which operates under a mixed market health care system, some physicians might voluntarily limit their practice to secondary care by requiring patients to see a primary care provider first, or this restriction may be imposed under the terms of the payment agreements in private/group health insurance plans. In other cases medical specialists may see patients without a referral, and patients may decide whether self- referral is preferred.

In the United Kingdom and Canada, patient self-referral to a medical specialist for secondary care is rare as prior referral from another physician (either a primary care physician or another specialist) is considered necessary; regardless of whether the funding is from private insurance schemes or national health insurance.

Allied health professionals, such as physical therapists, respiratory therapists, occupational therapists, speech therapists, and dietitians, also generally work in secondary care, accessed through either patient self-referral or through physician referral.

TERTIARY CARE

Tertiary care is specialized consultative health care, usually for inpatients and on referral from a primary or secondary health professional, in a facility that has personnel and facilities for advanced medical investigation and treatment, such as a tertiary referral hospital.

Examples of tertiary care services are cancer management, neurosurgery, cardiac surgery, plastic surgery, treatment for severe burns, advanced neo-natology services, palliative, and other complex medical and surgical interventions.

QUATERNARY CARE

The term quaternary care is sometimes used as an extension of tertiary care in reference to advanced levels of medicine which are highly specialized and not widely accessed. Experimental medicine and some types of uncommon diagnostic or surgical procedures are considered quaternary care. These services are usually only offered in a limited number of regional or national health care centres. This term is more prevalent in the United Kingdom, but just as applicable in the United States. A quaternary care hospital may have virtually any procedure available, whereas a tertiary care facility may not offer a sub-specialist with that training.

HOME AND COMMUNITY CARE

Many types of health care interventions are delivered outside of health facilities. They include many interventions of public health interest, such as food safety surveillance, distribution of condoms and needle-exchange programmes for the prevention of transmissible diseases. They also include the services of professionals in residential and community settings in support of self care, home care, long-term care, assisted living, treatment for substance use disorders and other types of health and social care services. Community rehabilitation services can assist with mobility and independence after loss of limbs or loss of function. This can include prosthesis, orthotics orwheelchairs.

Many countries, especially in the west are dealing with aging populations, and one of the priorities of the health care system is to help seniors live full, independent lives in the comfort of their own homes. There is an entire section of health care geared to providing seniors with help in day-to-day activities at home, transporting them to doctor's appointments, and many other activities that are so essential for their health and well-being. Although they provide home care for older adults in cooperation, family members and care workers may harbour diverging attitudes and values towards their joint efforts. This state of affairs presents a challenge for the design of ICT for home care.

With obesity in children rapidly becoming a major concern, health services often set up programmes in schools aimed at educating children in good eating habits; making physical education compulsory in school; and teaching young adolescents to have positive self-image.

HEALTH CARE INDUSTRY

The health care industry incorporates several sectors that are dedicated to providing health care services and products. As a basic framework for Classification categorizes health care as generally consisting of hospital activities, medical and dental practice activities, and "other human health activities". The last class involves activities of, or under the supervision of, nurses, midwives, physiotherapists, scientific or diagnostic laboratories, pathology clinics, residential health facilities, or other allied health professions, e.g. in the field of optometry, hydrotherapy, medical massage, yoga therapy, music therapy, occupational therapy, speech therapy, chiropody, homeopathy, chiropractics, acupuncture, etc. In addition, according to industry and market classifications, such as the Global Industry Classification Standard and the Industry Classification Benchmark, health care includes many categories of medical equipment, instruments and services as well as biotechnology, diagnostic laboratories and substances, and drug manufacturing and delivery. For example, pharmaceuticals and other medical devices are the leading high technology exports of Europe and the United States. The United States dominates the biopharmaceutical field, accounting for three-quarters of the world's biotechnology revenues.

HEALTH CARE FINANCING

There are generally five primary methods of funding health care systems:

1. general taxation to the state, county or municipality
2. social health insurance
3. voluntary or private health insurance
4. out-of-pocket payments
5. donations to health charities

In most countries, the financing of health care services features a mix of all five models, but the exact distribution varies across countries and over time within countries. In all countries and jurisdictions, there are many topics in the politics and evidence that can influence the decision of a government, private sector business or other group to adopt a specific health policy regarding the financing structure. For example, social health insurance is where a nation's entire population is eligible for health care coverage, and this coverage and the services provided are regulated. In almost every jurisdiction with a government-funded health care system, a parallel private, and usually for-profit, system is allowed to operate. This is sometimes referred to as two-tier health care or universal health care.

PRACTICE CONDITIONS AND REGULATIONS

SHORTAGES OF HEALTH PROFESSIONALS

Many jurisdictions report shortfalls in the number of trained health human resources to meet population health needs and/or service delivery targets, especially in medically underserved areas. For example, in the United States, the 2010 federal budget invested $330 million to increase the number of doctors, nurses, and dentists practising in areas of the country experiencing shortages of health professionals.

The Budget expands loan repayment programmes for physicians, nurses, and dentists who agree to practice in medically underserved areas. This funding will enhance the capacity of nursing schools to increase the number of nurses. It will also allow states to increase access to oral health care through dental workforce development grants. The Budget's new resources will sustain the expansion of the health care workforce funded in the Recovery Act.

In Canada, the 2011 federal budget announced a Canada Student Loan forgiveness programme to encourage and support new family physicians, nurse practitioners and nurses to practise in underserved rural or remote communities of the country, including communities that provide health services to First Nations and Inuit populations.

In Uganda, the Ministry of Health reports that as many as 50% of staffing positions for health workers in rural and underserved areas remain vacant. As of early 2011, the Ministry was conducting research and costing analyses to determine the most appropriate attraction and retention packages for medical officers, nursing officers, pharmacists, and laboratory technicians in the country's rural areas.

At the international level, the World Health Organization estimates a shortage of almost 4.3 million doctors, midwives, nurses, and support workers worldwide to meet target coverage levels of essential primary health care interventions. The shortage is reported most severe in 57 of the poorest countries, especially in sub-Saharan Africa.

HEALTH AND STRESS AMONG HEALTH CARE PRACTITIONERS

Some studies suggest that workplace stress is pervasive in the health care industry because of inadequate staffing levels, long work hours, exposure to infectious diseases and hazardous substances leading to illness or death, and in some countries threat of malpractice litigation. According to a report from the United States' National Institute for Occupational

Safety and Health, "health care workers have higher rates of substance abuse and suicide than other professions and elevated rates of depression and anxiety linked to job stress."

Elevated levels of stress were also linked to high rates of burnout, absenteeism and diagnostic errors, and to reduced rates of patient satisfaction. In Canada, a national report Canada's Health Care Providers also indicated higher rates of absenteeism due to illness or disability among health care workers compared to the rest of the working population, although those working in health care reported similar levels of good health and fewer reports of being injured at work.

According to the World Health Organization, women predominate in the formal health workforce in many countries, and are prone to musculoskeletal injury (caused by physically demanding job tasks such as lifting and moving patients) and burnout. Female health workers are exposed to hazardous drugs and chemicals in the workplace which may cause adverse reproductive outcomes such as spontaneous abortion and congenital malformations. In some contexts, female health workers are also subject to gender-based violence including from coworkers and patients.

Violence in the workplace subjects almost every health care worker to higher risk of on-the-job injury. Drunk, confused, and hostile patients and visitors are a continual threat to providers attempting to treat patients. Frequently, assault and violence in a health care setting goes unreported and is wrongly assumed to be part of the job.

PRACTISING WITHOUT A LICENSE

Practising without a license that is valid and current is typically illegal. In most jurisdictions, the provision of health care services is regulated by government, and individuals found to be providing medical, nursing or other professional services without the appropriate certification or licence may face sanctions including even criminal charges leading to prison. The number of professions subject to regulation, requisites for individuals to receive professional licensure, and nature of sanctions that can be imposed for failure to comply vary across jurisdictions.For instance, in the United States, under Michigan state laws, an individual is guilty of a felony if found to be practising a health profession subject to regulation without a valid license or registration of their own, or exceeding what a limited license or registration allows. The state laws define the scope of practice for medicine, nursing, and a number of allied health professions. In Florida, practising medicine without the appropriate license is a crime classified as a third degree felony, which may give imprisonment up to five years.

Practising a health care profession without a license which results in serious bodily injury classifies as a second degree felony, providing up to 15 years' imprisonment. In the United Kingdom, health care professionals are regulated by the state; the UK Health Professions Council (HPC) protects the 'title' of each profession it regulates. For example, it is illegal for someone to call themself an Occupational Therapist or Radiographer if they are not on the register held by the HPC.

APPLICATIONS IN HEALTH CARE

As well as seeking to improve population health through the implementation of specific population-level interventions, public health contributes to medical care by identifying and assessing population needs for health care services, including:

- Assessing current services and evaluating whether they are meeting the objectives of the health care system.
- Ascertaining requirements as expressed by health professionals, the public and other stakeholders.
- Identifying the most appropriate interventions.
- Considering the effect on resources for proposed interventions and assessing their cost-effectiveness.
- Supporting decision making in health care and planning health services including any necessary changes.
- Informing, educating, and empowering people about health issues.

IMPLEMENTING EFFECTIVE IMPROVEMENT STRATEGIES

To improve public health, one important strategy is to promote modern medicine and scientific neutrality to drive the public health policy and campaign, which is recommended by Armanda Solorzana, through a case study of the Rockefeller Foundation's hookworm campaign in Mexico in the 1920s. Soloranza argues that public health policy can't concern only politics or economics. Political concerns can lead government officials to hide the real numbers of people affected by disease in their regions, such as upcoming elections. Therefore, scientific neutrality in making public health policy is critical; it can ensure treatment needs are met regardless of political and economic conditions.

The history of public health care clearly shows the global effort to improve health care for all. However, in modern day medicine, real, measurable change has not been clearly seen, and critics argue that this lack of improvement is due to ineffective methods that are being implemented. As argued by Paul E. Farmer, structural interventions could possibly have a large impact, and yet there are numerous problems as to why this strategy has yet to be incorporated into the health system. One of the main reasons that he suggests could be the fact that physicians are not properly trained to carry out structural interventions, meaning that the ground level health care professionals cannot implement these improvements.

While structural interventions can not be the only area for improvement, the lack of coordination between socioeconomic factors and health care for the poor could be counterproductive, and end up causing greater inequity between the health care services received by the rich and by the poor. Unless health care is no longer treated as a commodity, global public health can ultimately not be achieved. This being said, without changing the way in which health care is delivered to those who have less access to it, the universal goal of public health care cannot be achieved.

❐

Chapter - 2

Quality Management for Health Care Delivery

INTRODUCTION

For the past 10 years American health policy has slowly shifted focus among three areas: access, cost, and quality of medical care. Each area has successively received concentrated attention, often at the expense of the other two. The situation can be viewed as a slowly rotating triangle that sequentially brings one after another of its vertices into principal focus. For example, access to care received primary attention during the late 1960's and early 1970s. That period saw the implementation of major federal initiatives intended to guarantee that all Americans could easily obtain high-quality health care. Medicare and Medicaid were introduced, a major national programme for mental health that reached into almost every community in the nation was instituted, and hospitals and medical schools were given federal monies for health care and health education programmes of every description. But during the late 1970s the federal government and private health financiers (principally industry) noted the high and increasing costs that grew from earlier 'access to care' initiatives.

The triangle turned. Emphasis shifted from a primary focus on access to a primary focus on cost. Federal programmes, such as the DRG prospective pricing system for Medicare, were developed to transfer financial risk to hospitals, introduce competition among health care providers, and contain the federal government's rising health care expenditures. Private insurers reacted with similar payment limitations to stop hospitals from shifting the resulting income shortfalls to their sector. Cost control efforts are now being extended to physicians as well as hospitals. It is not yet clear whether health care costs have been controlled. But financial risk sharing and competition have placed providers— physicians and hospitals—in an uncomfortable deliver, but that may simultaneously reduce access and quality. For many providers, cost controls are a matter not of declining profits but of financial survival. A growing chorus of providers, consumers, and political leaders voice a fear that, due to cost controls, needed care is being withheld. Recent research has solidified that fear by showing a close statistical association between stringent cost controls and high mortality rates. Anecdotes of cost-driven, low quality care abound.

The triangle is changing—it may no longer be acceptable to concentrate primary attention on a single vertex. Cost containment still demands close attention but quality and access are becoming simultaneous, serious concerns. The value of health care the highest possible quality at the lowest reasonable cost-is shifting into primary focus. But what is quality in health care? What is the relationship between quality and cost? Can health care costs be controlled only by sacrificing quality and access to care? How can a provider consistently achieve high quality care while meeting cost control constraints.? Continuous quality improvement (CQI) is a general theory for quality in any organized endeavor. It was originally set forth as a formal model in the 1930s by Walter A. Shewhart, an American engineer, and later expanded and refined by W. Edwards Deming and J. M. Juran. It has been widely applied to industry in Japan, where it is credited with that country's competitive success.

It is now appearing in industrial settings throughout the United States and Western Europe. Within the industrial setting it is generally called Industrial Quality Control, the industrial model for quality control, or total quality management-even though it is a broad range of ideas and techniques and often appears with different specific features in different industrial settings. Upon examination, medical applications of CQI theory predate Shewhart by many years. The roots of continuous quality improvement are the same quality principles that medical practice has taught since its inception. The major difference is that CQI theory uses those principles in a formal, explicit fashion. It rigourously applies the scientific method to organized medicine's commitment to 'learn from every patient, so that the next patient will receive better treatment'. Health care is significantly different from other industries. It is therefore not surprising that CQI systems designed for health care have features and emphases that are significantly different from those typically found in industrial quality control. CQI theory is important in the medical setting because it :

- Gives a rational definition of quality that applies in all health care settings,
- Clearly shows the relationship between health care costs and quality, and
- Leads to a system under which the highest quality care can consistently be delivered at the lowest justifiable cost.

The following chapters outline an application of CQI principles to health care. They proceed through five sections: the first introduces a consistent, generally applicable, description of health care quality; the second describes the relationship between quality and cost; the third outlines a system through which quality and cost can be scientifically evaluated, controlled, and documented; the fourth shows how CQI builds on the foundation of existing traditional quality assessment (QA) techniques; and the fifth presents a research model of health care to show that CQI principles offer opportunities for quality improvement and cost savings in every area of health care.

WHAT IS QUALITY?

In his classic text on health care quality Avedis Donabedian, M.D., presents a fundamental concept regarding the nature of any activity designed to produce a consistent result." Such an activity has three components:

- Structure → Process → Outcome

  The Process component may itself be regarded as consisting of.
- Input → Action → Output

More concretely, the practice of medicine is a process that results in an output. It is not the output alone. "Quality of production" refers to the process; "quality of design," or "quality of output, describes the end product. The "quality" of an output is an evaluation—an individual's personal judgement—of some set of attributes of the output. It is formed from the individual's perceptions of the output and is rooted within the individual's personal frame of reference. It is a relative term with no fixed unit of measurement, that is, a unitless value system. It is assessed by comparison to other similar items or events, so that static terms of "good quality" or "bad quality," as fixed measures, have no firm meaning over time—there is really only "better quality" or "worse quality."

The basis for comparison is contained within the individual's past personal experiences and prejudices. This personal history is expressed as expectations: when positive expectations are met, then quality is judged to be acceptable; when expectations are exceeded then quality is judged to be excellent. It is important to note that, more than being a unitless measure, "quality" is not a physical attribute of the service or product—it does not exist until there is an interaction between the product or service and the person making the judgement. Quality is thus a perception that is based on an individual's value system.

It relies heavily on the culture, life experiences, and expectations of each individual. Quality receives a new definition in each interaction between an individual and an item for which the term is evaluated. It is "one of those things that is very difficult to define, but that anyone can recognize-I know it when I see it." A prominent feature of unitless value systems is that, while they may be described, it is extremely difficult to mandate an a priori value standard that will be functionally acceptable to most people. A number of modern philosophers have noted that organizations (such as governments and health systems) operate under an umbrella of values that are generated by the culture of the society in which they exist.

While governments and organizations may be able to identify particular quality-based value systems, and even to influence them over long periods of time through education, they are not able to dictate fixed standards for quality that will be acceptable to all or even most individuals who relate to the organization. Individuals bring quality expectations to the organization—the organization does not tell the individuals what their quality values will be. And, as value systems depend upon a particular individual at a particular time, they are in a state of constant change and re-expression; they represent a moving target. When an organization or individual generates outputs, either as products or services, and delivers those outputs to other organizations or individuals, then a quality judgement can occur.

A customer is any organization or individual who makes quality judgements about, or has expectations regarding, an output. Although it is impossible to mandate quality expectations, it is possible to:

- Explicitly identify customer groups,
- Explicitly measure their expectations, and
- Change their expectations over time, through customer education.

In this setting, quality is meeting or exceeding customers' expectations 100 percent of the time. But customer expectations continually change. The definition of quality can therefore be expanded as follows:

- High quality is achieved by continual improvement in terms of customers' expectations. The aim of continuous quality improvement is to meet the customer, not just the competition.

Health care delivery is a complicated process which involves large numbers of workers. Different workers have different customers, depending upon the nature of an individual worker's job assignment. While, by definition, different customers have different expectations, they can be grouped together—general classes of customer expectations can be formed.

IDENTIFYING CUSTOMERS

Every division within a hospital has a different set of customer groups. For example (in very general terms), the hospital's primary customers may include patients and their families, secondary care physicians, payers, primary care physicians, employees, regulators, and local communities. A secondary care physician's customers could include patients and their families, primary care physicians who refer patients for care, the hospital administration, and payers. The laundry department's customers might include acute care nursing floors, surgery, and the maintenance department. The important concepts are the following:

- Any person or organization who has expectations regarding outputs is, by definition, a customer. Almost everyone—even suppliers— can profitably be treated as customers.
- Different hospital workers have different customers, including internal customers—individuals or departments within the hospital who use the worker's outputs.
- It is therefore necessary for every worker to understand the concept of "customers." They must be able to identify, and should explicitly list, their customers. The list should regularly be reviewed and updated.
- Individual customers can often be grouped together on the basis of similar needs and expectations.
- As will be detailed later in this report, supervisors and managers should not be their employees' primary customer—such a situation is the hallmark of poor management.

MEDICAL CUSTOMERS: CONTENT AND DELIVERY

Customer expectations can be divided into two major areas: expectations regarding the physical attributes, or content, of the output/product that is provided, and expectations about the nature of the interaction between the producer and the customer as the transaction takes place. Content quality refers to whether the output does what the customer believes it should do—does the output functionally meet the customer's expectations? Delivery quality refers to all aspects of the organization's interaction with the customer in delivering the output. It is determined day by day, moment by moment, in thousands of individual, temporary relationships. Does the customer's interaction with the organization's employees meet the customer's expectations? Within hospital- based health care delivery, content quality is roughly equivalent to medical outcomes.

Did the patient receive the medical out come that should have been achieved? Delivery quality describes, in a general way, patients' satisfaction with their hospital experiences. Neither distinction has clear boundaries: content and delivery quality interact extensively. But the dichotomy is useful for understanding and analyzing health care quality. As was mentioned in the Introduction, health care delivery is different from other industries. A major source of that difference is medicine's traditional approach to content quality: Medicine is one of the "learned professions." As such, it reserves to itself the right to judge its own quality. In functional terms, that means that the medical profession, as a group, sets its own expectations regarding medical outcomes (content quality)—a profession is sometimes its own primary customer. Medical outcome expectations are set by informal consensus as expressed in the medical literature and local "standards of care." Wennberg has written of the clinical hypothesis which underlies all diagnostic and treatment decisions. A clinical hypothesis describes the disease process, treatment options, and likely outcomes that can be achieved by different treatment strategies within traditional medical practice. Clinical hypotheses are usually not explicitly written out. But, in most instances, there is little debate regarding the outcomes that medical professionals hope a treatment will achieve. The medical profession's hold over medical content quality is beginning to erode. Patients and payers are becoming more informed and taking a more active part in setting medical outcome expectations. However, medical professionals still play the central rote. Nearly all patients and payers still to malpractice litigation. A second, related, major difference between health care delivery and other industries is medicine's opportunity for customer education.

EDUCATING PATIENTS

Hospitalization is a rare experience for most Americans. Their expectations regarding medical outcomes are often poorly defined, arising from television and the experiences of friends and relatives. The health care industry therefore has a greater opportunity than most other industries: through patient education, expectations can be set at the time the patient enters the hospital. In fact, that is exactly what happens in traditional medical practice. But patient (and family) education is often informal, uneven, and incomplete—it is frequently accomplished as a side thought to the 'real' business of medical treatment. But patient satisfaction has been shown to relate directly to how well the health care team informed the patient and family of the disease process and its treatment and whether the patient and family were allowed to participate in treatment decisions.

Both of these factors are functions of patient education. Said another way, many patients are frightened and confused by their illness and the medical interventions that are employed. They do not know how to interpret sensations in their own bodies and the actions of those in whose hands they have placed their lives. The sutures closing their surgical wound feel like they could tear loose if they cough. Will that happen? Their IV seems to be running more slowly. Does it need to be immediately adjusted? When they call the nurse, why is s/he so long in coming? Through education, patients are taught what is and is not important in their own condition. They become active members of the health care team.

Their anxiety decreases. They can join in treatment decisions. Their satisfaction with the health care system improves. For example, an Intermountain Health Care QUE (for Quality, Utilization, and Efficiency) study on non-acute cholecystectomy detected a physician whose patients left the hospital much earlier than did his colleagues' patients, while achieving comparable medical outcomes. That physician used a subcostal incision to reduce post-surgical pain, so that only non-narcotic analgesics were required for pain control. His patients regained bowel function more rapidly and so could be discharged earlier—on the average, within one or two days after surgery. Presented with these data, his colleagues supported his clinical approach, but asserted that patients could not comfortably assume their own care so early and so must be very dissatisfied with the care they had received. But on review it was found that his patients were among the most satisfied in the study.

The difference was patient education. The physician had prepared a videotape that stepped each patient through the events of their coming surgery. They were taught about factors that could be safely ignored and about those for which they should immediately seek help. Finally, they were told that they would recover just as quickly at home and that, with proper home care, they would be just as safe and even more comfortable. Another branch of patient education is important for risk management: Wennberg has investigated the use of interactive video disks to obtain informed consent for elective surgical procedures. Their use not only educates the patient, but documents the information that was given. Defects in informed consent form the basis for a significant proportion of malpractice actions against hospitals. Better patient education and informed consent could reduce that number.

QUALITY AND COST

Walter A. Shewhart, the father of formal continuous quality improvement theory, noted that "Price has no meaning without a measure of the quality being purchased." Quality and cost are intimately related: value is the combination of the quality of a product and the cost at which that level of quality is achieved. When discussing the cost and quality of clinical treatments (the content of care, as opposed to its delivery) that definition can be limited:

- High value clinical care results from the most efficient expenditure of resources to achieve an established high level of clinical quality.

Health care financiers—as represented by those industrial managers who are responsible for workers' health care benefits—have identified the value of health care as their principal focus over the next several years. They want to stop the steady upward pressure of health care costs while maintaining the best possible clinical quality, as reflected by clinical outcomes. Most health care practitioners would agree that costs and quality are inextricably intertwined, but CQI theory takes an extra step that some practitioners might find counter- intuitive: it asserts that high quality can lead directly to lower costs. To demonstrate the boundaries of that effect, the following paragraphs divide the relationship of cost and quality into five major areas:

- Quality waste,
- Productivity,
- Maximalism versus optimalism in the face of limited resources,
- The effect of improving the best medical outcome that can be achieved through new technology, new medications, or new techniques, and
- Environmental factors and the role of preventive medicine.

QUALITY WASTE

As part of the definition of quality developed in the previous section, Donabedian's fundamental quality model-processes that convert inputs into outputs-was introduced. But what happens if a process fails, and an output that does not meet quality expectations is produced? By definition, the output is a quality failure. Two options are available to deal with the offending product:

- Throw it away or
- Fix it.

Within non-health care industries these two options are called, respectively, scrap and rework. For service industries (including the delivery side of health care), scrap corresponds to abandoning a customer before the commissioned service has been satisfactorily performed, while rework takes the form of field service repairmen and customer service representatives. For medical outcomes— content quality—scrap and rework manifest themselves as mortality, morbidity, and the extra medical resources expended in attempts to correct bad outcomes. The low quality that results when a process fails brings with it a series of high costs. When a unit of output is scrapped, all of the resources that went into its production are wasted. Who pays for the scrapped units?

When a unit of output is repaired, additional resources must be allocated to correct the deficiency. Who pays for the repair work? Even more resources are consumed to replace customers (who cease to do business with the organization because they are dissatisfied with the quality of the output they received), in additional warranty costs (the organization may be liable for legal expenses and other, secondary damages that are traced to the original failure), and in time spent by managers who must deal with dissatisfied customers. Low quality leads directly to higher costs. These costs, arising from an initial process failure and the resulting low quality output, are termed quality waste. Quality waste represents the resources that are consumed, in the form of scrap or repairs, when a unit of output fails to meet quality expectations.

Quality waste can be traced by identifying scrap and rework. It can then be managed and eliminated from within an organization. Continuous quality improvement experts have measured quality waste in other (non-medical) industries. When a welt-managed quality control system was not in place, quality waste was consistently found to account for a significant proportion of the company's total dollar volume. As quality waste was recognized the companies involved made substantial gains in cost control and profitability. Based on conversations with quality leaders from large American health care systems, quality waste also exists in health care delivery. As it is discovered and corrected, quality can be improved and costs lowered. Three examples follow.

QUALITY WASTE IN HOSPITAL MANAGEMENT

When a service function fails repair takes the form of customer service representatives. One service that a hospital performs is patient billing. The bill's goal is to induce the patient to send payment. Bills are sent to patients so that the patient can relate the items for which they must pay to he services they actually received in the hospital. A bill should therefore accurately and completely list the services that were performed and the products that were used in a manner that the patient can understand and relate to their recent experience in the hospital. The billing process used by a 500-bed tertiary-care hospital failed to meet these simple criteria. Line items on detailed patient billing statements were so obtuse that even attending physicians could not understand them. A significant proportion of patients called with questions and complaints about bills. The hospital eventually hired a total of 12 full- time customer service representatives to deal with billing complaints alone. Direct costs for this repair activity were more than $300,000 per year. Moreover, hospital administrators spent significant amounts of their time answering patient complaints about bills, and many patients were known to take their health care needs to other providers because of their negative experience with the billing system. These expenditures all represent the costs of a failed process and a low quality output: they are quality waste. The concept can be summarized by a single basic precept of continuous quality improvement.

Do it Right the First Time

The hospital is now restructuring its patient bills. Physicians and patients helped plan the new billing system to guarantee that customers' needs will he met. The hospital stands to realize substantial savings as its need for customer service representatives declines.

CLINICAL QUALITY WASTE - I

Small area variation analysis examines differences in rates of hospitalization or the use of specific surgical procedures across small geographic districts. John Wennberg, M.D., pioneered the methodology through his analysis of the rates at which transurethral prostatectomies (TURPs) were performed in communities in Maine. He discovered that the procedure was performed at widely different rates in different communities, and that those differences could not be explained by variation in the underlying population. A "clinical hypothesis" is the set of available medical knowledge about a disease process, treatment options, and the medical outcomes likely to result from each treatment option.

Clinical hypotheses are usually implicit in medical practice—they are very rarely explicitly written out—but there is little disagreement among practitioners regarding their chief features and endpoints. Part of the clinical hypothesis for benign prostatic hypertrophy (BPH—the condition for which most TURPs are employed) concerned the natural history of the disease. Physicians know that many men develop BPH during their sixth or seventh decades of life, but only a fraction will eventually develop severe disease leading to urethral obstruction that requires surgical intervention. But they also know that, as men become older and more debilitated, the risks of any surgical procedure increase. Some physicians in Maine believed, as part of the BPH clinical hypothesis, that it was better to operate on a large group of men when they were relatively young—in their early sixties—than to operate on a smaller population of older men after their BPH became more severe. They thought there were fewer total deaths by pursuing the earlier, more vigourous surgical course. Wennberg demonstrated that the unwritten clinical hypothesis was wrong.

He showed that the death rate from surgical complications was much higher than expected, and that the risks of early surgery in a large population far outweighed the risks of age and advanced urethral obstruction in a smaller population of older patients. Upon publication of his results, the rate at which TURPs were performed in Maine felt precipitously. Fewer procedures were performed at a tower total cost, while the general quality of health care improved because many patients weren't exposed to the unnecessary risks of the procedure. By definition, a flawed clinical hypothesis means that either poor medical outcomes will be obtained or that the outcomes that are obtained will be relatively valueless. A flawed clinical hypothesis is therefore an excellent example of quality waste. Wennberg identified over 60 additional surgical procedures and medical diagnoses which exhibit similar regional variation. He has shown that such geographic variation can be a sign of a flawed clinical hypothesis. There is tremendous potential to improve the overall quality of medical care and reduce health care costs by studying and improving clinical hypotheses.

CLINICAL QUALITY WASTE II

Postoperative deep wound infections are an important cause of mortality and morbidity—low-quality outcomes—among surgical patients. Antibiotic prophylaxis is one useful step in a process designed to prevent such outcome failures. Members of the department of Infectious Disease at LDS Hospital, a 520 bed tertiary care teaching and referral center in Salt Lake City, Utah, prospectively monitored prophylactic antibiotic usage for all inpatient elective surgeries performed at their hospital during two six-month periods. They wanted to detect output failures (deep wound infections) and relate their occurrence to the process of care. All elective surgical cases that were admitted from June to November during 1985 or 1986 and that received antibiotic prophylaxis were monitored (4,484 cases). The timing of administration of the antibiotic was recorded: Prophylaxis was termed 'premature,' 'optimal,' or 'late' if the drug was given more than two hours before surgical incision time, within two hours before surgical incision time, or after surgical incision time, respectively.

Cases were identified and followed through the HELP Hospital Information System, a complete electronic medical record system developed at LDS Hospital. Baseline data were collected during the 1985 phase of the study. Then, during the first six months of 1986, steps were taken to modify the process by which prophylactic antibiotics were used at LDS Hospital: The HELP system was programmed to automatically evaluate each new elective surgery patient then insert a reminder that emphasized the two-hour ,optimal' time period in the patient's electronic medical record. Copies of the reminder were also printed and attached to the patient's chart. All eligible patients were again prospectively monitored from June to November 1986, under the new reminder system. The total percentage of patients who received antibiotic prophylaxis did not change.

But the percentage of patients receiving prophylaxis during 'optimal' times increased significantly, rising from 40 percent in 1985 to 58 percent in 1986 ($P< 0.001$). This was associated with a decline in deep post-operative wound infections from 1.8 percent (28 infections) to 0.9 percent (16 infections; $p < 0.03$). The deep wound infections found in the study required extended hospitalization and treatment. They ranged from relatively simple, easily manageable, infections of abdominal incisions (e.g., following an appendectomy) to life-threatening deep infections of the mediastinum following open-heart surgery. LDS Hospital spends, on average, between

$13,000 and $15,000 to treat every deep wound infection that occurs within its walls. A partial correction of the process of giving prophylactic antibiotics at the hospital reduced the number of infections during the six-month period from 32 expected cases to 16 actual cases. The 16 cases in which infections were avoided translates to a cost savings, for the hospital, insurers, and patients, of over $400,000 per year in fixed costs alone. In addition, postoperative infections may expose the attending physician and hospital to legal action. Most important, such infections can cause permanent damage to a patient and may result in a preventable death.

PRODUCTIVITY

Suppose that two different processes start with identical inputs and produce identical outputs, but that one uses twice as many resources as the other. Which process should be used? A number of studies have documented the broad range of practice patterns, and widely varying resource consumption, that are employed by practitioners to achieve apparently identical clinical results. Donabedian notes that, when total health resources are limited, inefficient practice styles do positive quality harm: wasted resources cannot be used to meet the legitimate needs of other patients. In an era of limited medical resources—as evidenced by medical cost containment efforts and serious questions regarding access to care—suboptimal practice patterns are clearly unacceptable.

IHC QUE STUDIES

Both the hospital and its physicians have major impacts on the nature of care that is delivered within a hospital. Researchers at intermountain Health Care in Salt Lake City, Utah, developed a model that separates the hospital's contribution from physicians' contributions to clinical care. The QUE model (for Quality, Utilization, and Efficiency) focuses on "units of care." Units of care correspond to the individual items on a detailed patient bill—for example, a single dose of a drug, one minute in a surgical suite, or one day on an acute care nursing floor. The hospital is regarded as a factory that produces units of care. The efficiency with which the hospital produces each unit of care, as reflected in true unit costs,* can be examined. Physicians then combine varying numbers of different units of care into a health care product. Physician utilization patterns, as expressed in numbers of specific units of care employed, can be analyzed.

But before either utilization or efficiency can be examined it is necessary to form a balanced group of patients who had equal -acuity (severity of illness), complexity (presence and severity of comorbidities), and out comes (complications and medical results). These factors are jointly viewed as quality. The aim of an IHC QUE study is to compare and contrast physicians (in terms of utilization) and hospitals (in terms of efficiency), with a view to identify and eliminate inappropriate variation. It requires a team approach. While a QUE study can document variation it cannot determine whether the variation is appropriate or inappropriate. A QUE study's blinded results are therefore reported to the hospitals and physicians involved to act upon as they deem best.

A major precept of CQI theory states that most individuals-85 to 90 percent-pursue high-quality work as a personal value; it is only necessary to supply adequate data and training to achieve high-quality results. This may be even more true in clinical medicine, which tends to attract those with a personal commitment to serve. IHC has completed QUE studies for six clinical entities. Very high variation was observed from physician to physician (in terms of utilization) and from hospital to hospital (in terms of efficiency) for every clinical area examined. Nine months after utilization variation data for TURPs were shown to physicians at three hospitals, a follow-up TURP QUE Study was conducted to determine if the original findings had had any impact. The only action taken following the first study was to confidentially share variation data with individual physicians. More important, the amount of variation from physician to physician also declined for most major units of care. The second principle of quality management states: to achieve high quality, eliminate inappropriate variation, Inappropriate variation—in this case, variation that increases costs but does not lead to improved medical outcomes—is a hallmark of low productivity. When differences in the processes that lead to apparently identical medical outcomes are identified, three possibilities exist:

- Some practitioners are under-utilizing and run an increased risk for quality failures,
- Some practitioners are over-utilizing and use resources that aren't really required, or

- There are differences in skills and clinical acumen among the practitioners—some physicians require more resources to achieve the same output. In the first case, utilization should be appropriately increased.

In the second, it may be appropriately decreased. In the final case, the underlying variation clearly is not inappropriate, although recognition of this situation can lead to additional training and improvement in clinical skills.

OPTIMALISTS AND MAXIMALISTS

Quality waste represents the process failures in medical care, their inherent low quality, and the high costs required to repair them. Low productivity— the use of techniques that are not as cost effective to achieve an equivalent output—is harmful by displacing more effective care. It is believed that as one adds to the total care delivered for a particular episode of illness, the marginal content qualityachieved by each additional unit of care declines. In the extreme, marginal quality gains become trivially small while costs rise without limit. A point may be reached where the gains in quality cannot justify the in creased consumption of limited medical resources. Those who hold this view may be called optimalists," as they attempt to achieve an optimal level of quality achieved for resources consumed (that is, they try to maximize value). The main potential harm resulting from optimalism is that while a very high level of quality may be achieved, the ultimate pinnacle of potential content quality for an individual patient may not be reached.

A second view holds that, from an ethical standpoint, health care professionals cannot be placed in the position of limiting medical content quality on the basis of cost. The best possible medical output should always be pursued, regardless of cost. Those who support this view are called "maximalists." As with low productivity, the principal harm engendered by maximalism is that, by consuming unlimited resources for limited gains, it potentially displaces more useful care. Maximalism differs from low productivity in that, by definition, low productivity occurs when an alternative approach will achieve the same quality using fewer resources; maximalism achieves higher quality but at an increasingly unfavorable cost.

Donabedian notes that health care practitioners tend to be maximalists because they then need only decide if an additional element of care will be useful. Optimal care requires added expertise regarding cost and some method of balancing the usefulness of each additional element of care against its cost. In fact, traditional American medical practice has long included a strong dose of optimalism—it is legitimate, ethical, and even necessary when limited medical resources must be allocated among unlimited medical demands, so long as the costs and benefits are jointly weighed by the health care professional and a fully informed patient. A much more difficult (and, often, ethically unacceptable) situation arises when a third party—typically a health care financier or regulator—independently establishes and then enforces a particular level of care as being optimal.

NEW TECHNOLOGY

The science and technology of medicine continue to rapidly advance. There is little question that improved technology, new pharmaceuticals, and updated therapeutic approaches provide a greater likelihood of a superior medical outcome. Government regulations require that new technology be demonstrated to be "effective and efficacious" before it can be distributed throughout the country. New techniques are demonstrated through clinical research and reported in the medical literature before they find widespread acceptance. New techniques and technology change the final output expectations for medical content. Such changes mean that the underlying process has been modified to produce a different, superior output. These improvements nearly always involve higher costs. At a fundament at level, significant improvements in the best final output that the process of medical care can hope to achieve consume more resources than their less capable predecessors. The optimalist/maximalist debate often intrudes in discussions of new technology. While existing techniques and technologies are somewhat protected by their traditional use, new innovations may be criticized on the basis of their perceived cost-benefit ratio. But the fact remains—some advances in medical care, which improve the best output that can he achieved, can be had only with the expenditure of more resources.

ENVIRONMENTAL FACTORS AND PREVENTIVE MEDICINE

Finally, the role of preventive medicine and environmental health in controlling the costs of medical care, while improving the overall quality of Americans' health, should not be overlooked. Environmental and personal lifestyle factors (e.g., air quality, toxic wastes, automobile trauma, and tobacco usage) have been shown to have a profound impact on the rates of disease within our communities and, thus, upon the total cost of medical care that society must bear.

As a related discipline, preventive medicine is generally recognized as being much more cost-effective than the treatment of established disease in achieving positive health outcomes. If one accepts the premise that there is a limited fund of health care resources from which essentially unlimited health care demands must be satisfied, then there is a strong incentive to eliminate those known environmental and lifestyle factors which lead to disease and consume large amounts of medical resources. Some of the harshest critics of American medicine's high costs— leaders in industry, government, and special interest groups—are in the best position to control medical costs by controlling those environmental and lifestyle factors that lead to disease.

A SYSTEM FOR CONTINUOUS QUALITY I MPROVEMENT AND COST CONTROL

Achieving high quality and appropriate cost reductions involves three major steps:

- prepare to improve,
- implement, and
- innovate.

Once a CQI system is in place, steps 2 and 3 cycle continuously. These steps can also be stated in CQI's two primary principles: To continuously improve quality and appropriately control costs, eliminate inappropriate variation and document continuous improvement. Their effective application depends upon a clear understanding of the nature of quality ("quality is meeting customer expectations"), the role of process in achieving quality, and the relationship between quality and cost. To "prepare to improve," steps 1 through 5 are all necessary in some form:

- Find a process. Health care is a complicated series of related processes. A large number of those processes are already well defined through clinical practice—individual diagnoses and procedures (health care products) each represent a process. Taken together they form the heart of health care delivery. Other processes cut across diagnostic lines. For example, admission to the hospital, billing, or analyzing a single blood test are all definable processes that cross diagnostic lines. The first step is to choose a process that needs quality improvement and cost control.
- Assemble a team that knows the process. Those who best understand a process are nearly always those who perform it on a daily basis— frontline workers. Through its members, the team must also have an understanding of continuous quality improvement principles, statistical quality control, the use of data management systems, and access to management so that organizational roadblocks to improvement can be overcome.
- Identify customers, identify process outputs, and measure customer expectations regarding the outputs. By definition, quality is meeting or exceeding the expectations held by a process's

customers (with the proviso that expectations can be changed, over time, through customer education). But different processes have different outputs and often have different customers. The team's first task is therefore to list the outputs of the process, identify its customers, and measure their expectations of its outputs. It is important that these steps be done explicitly—in writing. Too often American organizations have confused their customers' expectations with their own, internal expectations. Such quality standards are called measures of self- gratification- they soon degenerate into systems for making the company look good in its own eyes, instead of meeting customers' expectations and thus protecting the company's survival. The best way to avoid this trap is to explicitly list the process's customers and then measure their expectations. The customer list, output list, and expectation measurements should be updated from time to time; they are the foundation upon which the entire quality process is built. They can change as customer groups shift, the process evolves, and customers gain knowledge. Within clinical medicine, the customer is the medical profession as a whole. Its expectations are expressed through clinical hypotheses as defined in the preceding section. For clinical diagnoses or procedures, "measuring expectations" corresponds to discovering and writing down clinical hypotheses. Obviously, because clinical expectations are generated by the profession as a whole rather than by individual practitioners or hospitals, they can best be documented on a profession-wide scale.

- Document the process. A process consists of a series of steps that convert inputs into outputs. They are usually hierarchical; that is, the main process may be broken down into subprocesses, each with subinputs and suboutputs. Each of the resulting subprocesses may similarly be broken down into sub-subprocesses, again with sub- subinputs and sub-suboutputs. The hierarchical chain may be followed to that level of detail necessary to understand the process. Some elements in a process are associated with its outputs but do not actually cause them. Others are causal—their presence or absence determines whether an output or suboutput will have features that meet explicit expectations: key process factors (KPFs) are process steps that causally determine whether an output will meet quality expectations. The team must explicitly document—in written form— those KPFs that lead to the desired output: Fundamental (or substantive) knowledge describes the steps in a process and identifies its key process factors. Fundamental knowledge usually resides in front-line workers who deal with the process in a detailed manner on a daily basis. It leads to ideas about how the process can be changed and improved over time. A process cannot be managed without fundamental knowledge.

- Generate output and process specifications. A specification is an explicit, measurable, statement regarding an important attribute of an output(a customer expectation) or the (sub)process that produces it (key process factors). In Steps 3 and 5 above the team is charged to generate lists of customer expectations and KPFs. Those lists may be used to generate a list of specifications—statements regarding the output features that are to be produced and the process steps that will lead to them. Specifications define measurement variables. They make no statement about "acceptable" levels of achievement. Note that specifications are generated in two areas: external, customer expectations and internal, process expectations. They reflect both the goals that a process was created to achieve, and the manner in which those goals are planned to be accomplished. They must be stated so that they are explicitly measurable. Finally, they should be updated as customer expectations change and as the process is improved. Specifications are a necessary part of any process, whether managed through CQI or some other system. The only real question is whether they will be explicitly stated. If the specifications for a process or subprocess are not explicitly stated, then it is impossible to measure whether the process is consistently achieving its goals. Explicit specifications form the basis for an objective measurement system as well as providing opportunity for criticism of and improvements to the specifications themselves: Quality cannot be achieved without a sufficient set of measurable specifications that reflect customer expectations and key process factors. Specifications therefore provide the basis for managing quality. As they are framed in terms of customer expectations, they are the definition of "quality" for a process. That is, when specifications are property stated, achievement of the specifications is equivalent to achievement of quality. Much of the effort of a quality organization centers around producing suitable specifications and implementing effective measurement systems. If all of the necessary pieces are in place, then the achievement of quality reduces to a single principle: Quality is conformance to specifications. The fact that specifications are explicitly written means that they can be criticized and modified. They can—and should—be adjusted as the process is more clearly understood or the desired outputs, as measured through customer expectations, change.

- Eliminate inappropriate variation (Implement). Specifications define measurement points. Once specifications are in place, those data points can be recorded for every input/output that transits the process. The goal is to detect quality events (outcomes) in subprocesses and final outputs, then to relate them to variation in the performance of KPFs in the process. Were other major procedures performed or diagnoses treated during this hospitalization?
- Foley catheter management: Date / time Foley catheter was initially removed. Did the patient require recatheterization? If so, how many times, with date and time? Was the patient discharged with a Foley catheter in place? What type of Foley catheter and irrigation system was used?
- Short-term complications: Did the patient experience:
  - Excessive blood loss (requiring transfusion),
  - Atelectasis or pneumonia,
  - Thrombophlebitis,
  - Infection or fever,
  - Water intoxication, or
  - Other in-hospital complications?
- Laboratory: What lab tests were ordered? When were they ordered?
- Pathology: How much time elapsed from surgery until the pathology report was available in the chart?
- Outplacement: Discharge destination (home, nursing home, etc.). Who was available to help the patient with home care? Was they patient, or someone associated with the patient, able (physically and through adequate knowledge) to provide the necessary posthospital care?
- Long-term complications: Did the patient experience:
  - Impotence,
  - Incontinence,
  - Urethral contractures,
  - Death within one month of discharge ,
  - Readmission to the hospital within 30 days,
  - Recatheterization at the ER or physician's office, or
  - Other complications arising from the procedure after hospital discharge?
- Medical outcome: Were the patient's urinary symptoms corrected? Was the patient's functional status improved!

- Was the patient satisfied with his or her hospital stay, the manner in which the procedure was performed, and its final results?

Statistical quality control (SQC) is a methodology that separates random variation from specific variation. It offers a means by which specific variation may be identified and then removed, by eliminating performance variation at key steps in the process. It also prevents well-meaning but uninformed changes that waste effort and, potentially, damage the process. (CQI theory defines tampering as changes implemented in an attempt to correct random variation. By definition, such variation results from random noise in the system. It cannot be traced to a specific cause so attempts to "correct" it in the process will necessarily fail.) Within clinical medicine, CQI forms a natural basis for cooperation between hospitals and health care professionals: hospitals have the data to document variation, but only health care professionals can say what is appropriate. Hospitals and health professionals can consistently achieve high-quality care only by working as a team. The measurement systems used to eliminate inappropriate variation must be explicit. Experience has repeatedly shown that implicit systems—under which progress towards a goal is intuitively evaluated—are frequently tainted by the reviewers' (often unconscious) preference for a particular result. Quality improvement systems must he designed to reflect factual performance against written specifications. This axiom is reflected in a principle of quality management:

- Within an effective quality management programme, a goal without an explicit measurement system to document continuous progress towards that goal is meaningless. The goal of eliminating inappropriate variation is to create a stable system, a system in which all specific variation has been eliminated and only random variation remains.

SPECIFICATIONS AND STANDARDS

Successful medical CQI systems are nearly always built on the foundation of an excellent traditional quality assurance QA) system. Beyond its description of the relationship of cost to quality and its explicit approach to process (in addition to outcome) measurement, CQI's main contributions to traditional QA are a series of formal mechanisms to deal with situations that traditional QA leaders were forced to solve on an ad hoc basis. Most of those situations center around the difference between specifications (within CQI) and standards (within traditional QA).

INHERENT ARBITRARINESS

Most standards contain an unavoidable element that is inherently arbitrary. By using quality absolutes (0 percent failure or 100 percent success), CQI circumvents them. For example, many cardiac surgery programmes insist that their overall mortality rate be no more than 3 percent. But why is 3 percent acceptable? Why not 2 percent (as a quality manager might choose) or 4 percent (as a physician being "managed" might choose)? Some standards are based upon statistical measures generated from an index population. For example, a mortality standard could be set at 3 percent because that was the mean mortality rate for some collection of hospitals for which data were available. But what makes the average (or any statistical measure) an acceptable standard for "quality"? By definition, some hospitals had to have a rate better than the average. If that superior rate could be obtained why is any lower standard acceptable.? How good is "good enough?" The inherently arbitrary nature of most standards is reflected in the fact that it is often much easier to achieve agreement among medical professionals on specifications for a clinical process- the end results that a course of treatment is intended to achieve-than on standards for the same process.

INHERENT MISCLASSIFICATION

CQI avoids a two-level classification system with an inherent misclassification rate. Many standard-based systems exist to flag some cases or providers for intensive review. This approach forces QA managers to deal with three difficult issues:

- Standards sometimes flag "good" cases, or fail to flag "bad" cases;
- "Intensive review" may itself he regarded as a judgement (and a punishment); and
- Standard-based systems usually focus only on flagged cases (potential failures), so they fail to associate process data with outcome data on every case.

They can become a classic example of trying to "inspect" quality into a process after the failures have already occurred, as described in the last section.

For example, consider the following actual standard: "patients with head injuries, who require a cranial CAT scan, should receive that procedure within four hours of admission to the hospital." But some patients should receive a cranial CAT scan much sooner—even a three-hour delay might be inappropriate. A different, more complex, diagnosis may appropriately require a cranial CAT scan on the second day of hospitalization—the standard would incorrectly flag that case. Appropriate variation may sometimes lead a good provider to fall on the "bad" side of a standard. A standard may fail to detect inappropriate variation in other cases. Said another way, a standard fails to distinguish random causes from attributable (special) causes, as described in the previous section.

If a standard-based QA programme is not carefully administered, providers may be held responsible for random causes over which they have no control—the intensive examination that results from a flagged case may itself become the punishment. In the example given above, a provider may order a cranial CAT scan on every patient with head injuries, regardless of indications, in order to avoid being flagged and subjected to detailed examination. That is, a provider may erroneously modify his/her process in an attempt to remedy a random cause. But, by definition, a random cause cannot be corrected by tampering with the process. The only effect of tampering is to introduce more variation and damage the process. CQI theory shows that it does little good to identify quality failures if those failures are not traced to specific variation in the production process. That implies that the production process must be simultaneously monitored and that every case—not just failures— should be recorded. That viewpoint rejects the idea of measuring outputs to "flag" some cases for further review. Finally, a dichotomous scale is not appropriate for a large subset of quality data—semi-continuous or continuous scales are much more effective analytic tools. The chief reason for a dichotomous scale (that is, a standard) is to reduce the work load for quality evaluators. It reduces the amount of data that must be reviewed and makes it easier to classify cases and providers as "good" or "bad."

ARTIFICIAL FLOORS AND CEILINGS

CQI avoids artificial floors and ceilings. Most standards carry a subtle message that is very hard to dispel: by definition, a standard represents an "acceptable" level of performance. Therefore, once a standard has been met, the drive for further improvement can be greatly diminished. In other words, a standard can become an artificial quality floor or ceiling. Within CQI, the only floors and ceilings are quality absolutes-0 percent failures or 100 percent successes. In some circumstances standards must be employed. But in those cases there should be a standing procedure that they will be re-evaluated and adjusted on a regular basis, to avoid artificial floors and ceilings.

ACCURATE PRIMARY DATA

CQI generates more accurate primary data. Most standards form at the base of "acceptable" versus "unacceptable" flagging systems. Nearly all are associated with some sort of overt or covert punishment, he it as subtle as an intensive review process, loss of professional prestige, or failure to receive an incentive reward, or as blatant as loss of a provider contract or a professional license. At the same time, most providers generate some portion of the data upon which they are evaluated. As a result, it is not unusual to see consistent (but often subconscious) changes in patient classification and evaluation that favour the provider. That is, a classification system with subtle, inherent disincentives can lead to bad primary data even among conscientious providers. What started as a quality improvement system can devolve into a game of "beat the system." A good example is HCFA's recent mortality data release and some hospitals' reaction to it.. Within CQI the only acceptable standards are quality absolutes— 100 percent success or 0 percent failure. That view avoids some of the inherent operational difficulties that traditional standards have forced QA leaders to face. From a CQI perspective, any "standard" other than perfection leads to the following definition:

- A traditional standard measures the amount of "acceptable" waste, through quality failures, that is intentionally built into a system.

Not all traditional quality assurance programmes are excellent. A system that lacks a true dedication to quality can degenerate to finding "bad apples" and actually damage overall quality. An excellent article, by Donald Berwick, M.D., on that subject is included in the Recommended Readings. CQI recognizes that errors will occur. It differs in its response to them:

- It avoids artificial quality ceilings and bad data by relating outcome to process, and using specifications instead of standards.
- It objectively traces quality failures to process failures by measuring process factors as well as outcome factors for all cases, not just failures (that is, it analyzes as well as enumerates).
- It attempts to correct errors by fixing the process, not the people. It also must pay the price of better, more extensive data collection and requires the same intense dedication to quality that has allowed some traditional QA programmes to overcome the hurdles that standards can present.

AN OPERATIONAL MODEL FOR QUALITY IN HEALTH CARE

An operational model is useful for several reasons: It provides an explicit description of health care quality-because it is explicit, it can be criticized, updated, and improved. It can describe relationships between areas of medical quality assurance that experience teaches are useful, while highlighting other areas that may have been overlooked.

The question is not whether a model will be employed, but whether the model that is used will be explicitly stated—and so amenable to criticism and improvement—or implicitly accepted without conscious thought regarding its strengths and weaknesses. The foregoing discussion on the nature of quality and the relationship of quality to cost identified several areas of quality management. It noted medicine's unique division between delivery quality (as measured by patients' expectations) and content quality (as measured by health delivery professionals' expectations, acting on behalf of patients).

It also observed that the achievement of quality depends almost entirely on the systems that health care delivery employs, and thus on the management teams who oversee those health care delivery systems. Finally, a number of fundamental concepts of quality management, necessary parts of any successful quality control effort, were set forth.

Four areas provide the major divisions that form the highest level of the proposed model. Each is of primary importance to a different group within health care. Therefore, they are presented in the order of complication of presentation, saving the most complicated, and hence the lengthiest, for last. The four major divisions of the model are the following:

- Quality of Management
- Quality of Evaluation
- Quality of Service (Delivery Quality)
- Value of Care (Content Quality)

QUALITY OF ORGANIZATION/MANAGEMENT

Continuous quality improvement is rooted in the culture of a health care organization. It requires that all workers in the organization understand the same quality terms, speak the same quality language, and share the same quality vision. Further, the consistent achievement of high-quality outputs depends upon the processes that an organization employs. The organization's management team constructs and oversees those processes. Arguably, good management is the most important factor that determines whether an organization will succeed in continuous quality improvement. Earlier sections made the point that health care delivery is different from other industries, Therefore, Industrial Quality Control (IQC), which represents the application of CQI principles in industrial settings, often cannot be applied directly to health care. But the management theory used by CQI differs little whether it is viewed from the standpoint of industry or health care. Many IQC texts focus heavily on management theory. With minor modification, they can be applied directly to hospital management. A number of IQC/management theory texts are therefore included in the Recommended Readings list at the end of this report.

MEASUREMENT, SPECIFICATIONS, AND REPORTING

The organization that is managing quality has regular answers to two questions: Are we doing the right things (strategic quality)? Are we doing things right (system quality) ? Consistent, planned progress in any endeavor is usually a two-step process: One first establishes a goal (strategic focus), then one tries to move towards that goal (systems focus).

The primary quality goal is to meet reasonable customer expectations, as set forth through output and process specifications, 100 percent of the time. Consistent, planned improvements in quality therefore require two measurement systems. The first tracks the moving goal of customer expectations. The second measures movement in relationship to that goal, to show whether a particular effort brought one closer to the goal or moved one farther away. As customer expectations are reflected in hierarchical specifications, the act of measuring progress towards a quality goal is equivalent to measuring the output of a process vis a vis the specifications for that process. Organizations usually display a hierarchical structure. Specifications can mimic that hierarchical structure, so that each subcomponent has the requisite freedom to define its internal role and accomplish it goals, while meeting the organizational purpose of its existence.

This structure also recognizes the fact that, in most organizations, those at the lowest management level-on the front line of interaction with customers—are those who best understand the organization's processes, know best how to improve them, and are best able to implement effective change. Hierarchical specifications can also form the foundation of a consistent reporting system. By following the structure set forth in a complete set of hierarchical specifications, a measurement system can evaluate quality at every level of an organization with an appropriate level of detail. The hierarchical structure ensures that, as reports move up the organizational chain, they can be meaningfully combined to reflect quality goals set for each level of the organization. In a very real sense, a set of hierarchical specifications are a direct statement of what a health care entity hopes to achieve at each level of its organization, and the means by which progress towards those goals can be measured. This concept provides one of the more useful forms of the underlying quality principle: Quality is how well an organization accomplishes that which it says it intends to do. This implies that the organization knows what it intends to do:

- It knows who its customers are (in content, delivery, and other areas) and it measures their expectations
- It knows what its outputs/products are-they have been specified and are appropriately monitored on the basis of those specifications
- It understands the structures and processes that lead to its outputs— subprocesses and intermediate outputs are also specified and monitored
- It understands the nature of quality management.

Obviously, an organization's top management is responsible for explicitly establishing the organization's quality goals.

QUALITY MISSION STATEMENT

Management's first responsibility is to clearly establish the quality focus of the organization. This takes the form of a quality mission statement. It is a general statement defining the outputs the organization plans to produce. It is thus the top-level specification from which all other output specifications used within the organization will derive. In order to be fully useful, a quality mission statement should include the following features that relate directly to the organization's management function:

- Constancy of purpose. Quality is a function of the processes that exist within an organization. Its successful accomplishment is the keystone by which the entire organization will stand or fall. Success or failure in achieving quality is therefore first the responsibility of the organization's managers. It is directly determined by the processes that the managers create and the managers' ability to lead: It begins in the board room, not on the hospital ward. Quality requires a long-term, hands-on commitment from the top leaders in an organization.
- Dedication to continuous improvement. As noted above, quality is a moving target. An organization must be dedicated to constant change and improvement, starting with its internal systems and moving to the products and services it offers. Specifications bracket the target, so as the target moves the specifications will change.
- Focus on the customer. An organization depends for its continued existence on its ability to anticipate, educate, and serve its customers. "Customer" is used in a very broad sense—the successful organization is seen as serving and educating nearly all with whom it comes in contact. A hospital's customers include patients, physicians, health care financiers, internal departments, suppliers, and other outside groups.
- Understanding the service or product. The organization must understand the underlying nature of the service or product that is delivered, and the process that leads to its successful production (also sometimes called "substantive, or fundamental, knowledge").
- Measurement systems. The statement of a goal without an explicit measurement system to document progress towards that goal is meaningless. Within a quality-based organization, hierarchical specifications serve to define the measurement system and to

guarantee that quality reports can be meaning fully combined as they move upward through the management chain.

MANAGEMENT'S ROLE

High Quality Depends Primarily on Good Management, not Worker Motivation

In most instances workers within a health care system have inherent personal pride in the work they do. The achievement of a particular level of quality is more a result of the systems under which they work than a problem with commitment or motivation. Quality is a function of process. Process depends on the systems by which the organization operates. These systems are directly structured and controlled by management. Therefore, the starting place for quality in any organization is top management. Organizations that attempt to establish quality by focusing exclusively on the end product and front-line workers, while ignoring the underlying management systems and their critical impact on quality, will fail to achieve high quality and the full range of secondary cost benefits it brings over time CQI theory presents several principles regarding an organization's management and its role in quality:

- *Top-down process.* The establishment of quality in an organization is a top-down process. Quality should therefore be a major concern of the chief executive officer of the corporation. While a committee or some other officer may be assigned day-to-day oversight of specific quality-monitoring operations, the CEO should have a direct, day-to-day responsibility to manage that process.
- *Front-line focus.* A quality organization recognizes that most workers are motivated by pride in their job, and builds systems that allow them to express that pride in terms of high quality. It recognizes that front-line workers best understand the problems involved in serving customers and producing health care products. It recognizes that most workers are already motivated, and only need an outlet for their innovative ideas. Finally, it recognizes that attitudes held by employees regarding the organization are often transferred directly to customers as health care services are delivered. If an employee believes that the organization strongly supports high quality, then this viewpoint will be conveyed to the customers served by the employee. All workers in the organization:

- Should know that they can have a direct impact on the structure of the systems used by the organization (that is, their concerns will be promptly and competently addressed)
- Should not fear overt or covert reprisal for criticizing the systems used by the organization
- Should he encouraged by the structure and operation of the organization to be oriented to the needs of their true customers rather than to those of their supervisors

Ultimately, quality is delivered by the employee who builds the product or interacts with the customer. "At the interface" employees have the best understanding of customers' needs and expectations on an individual basis and are directly responsible for meeting them. The remaining structure of the organization—including management—exists to support front-line employees in their critical rote. Successful organizations find ways to stimulate, test, and implement the quality improvement ideas that their front-line employees generate.

They also recognize that every employee of the organization is, in one sense, a front-tine employee—it is just that managers work on the "front-line" of producing management systems, rather than the traditional products envisioned by the company's leaders. The same quality principles that apply to improvements in operational processes may also be applied to achieve improvements in management processes.

Management's principal tasks are to:

- Commit
  - Demonstrate constancy of purpose
  - Imbue the organization with a stable long-term strategic vision
  - Establish an organization-wide quality mission statement
  - Show top-down management commitment to quality in actions as well as words (quality starts with the board and CEO)
- Understand
  - Know the business of the company (sometimes called substantive or fundamental knowledge); management must have hands-on experience with the processes and products upon which the organization depends for its continued existence
  - Learn the following principles of quality measurement, and teach them throughout the organization:
  - Specification, data collection, and process measurement

  - The nature of random ("common") versus attributable ("specific") variation
  - Enumerative versus analytic techniques
- Identify
  - Customers, products, and processes (i.e., generate valid specifications)
- Educate and train
  - Employees, in their jobs and in quality principles
  - Customers (at all levels, as defined above), in order to guide their expectations
- Measure
  - Customer expectations, process outputs, and outcomes
- Manage
  - Eliminate quality waste
  - Increase productivity
- Test
  - Use the Shewhart cycle and front-line employees to constantly improve the organization's production and management processes
- Establish appropriate incentives
  - Most improvement is team based; reward teams, not individuals
  - Focus incentives on
    a. Reductions in quality waste and
    b. Tested and proven innovation
  - Eliminate incentives that reward behaviour that benefits an individual or a particular unit, but damages the organization as a whole
- Lead (rather than supervise)
  - Remove quality barriers
  - Empower front-line employees and always: Eliminate inappropriate variation and document continuous improvement.

Finally, Philip Crosby identified the following principle for quickly identifying high-quality management practices within an organization:

- What originally began as "quality" has now expanded with experience into an understanding that "hassle elimination" and "quality improvement" are the same.

QUALITY OF EVALUATION

Quality is a moving target. Its attainment is a function of process within an organization. It is therefore necessary to continually measure progress towards quality goals and to study the underlying processes of the business in order to encourage innovation and continual improvement. In order to effectively evaluate quality, management must understand the principles of random variation as they relate to quality.

Management must also be committed to the use of proper methodological toots to detect and then reduce the inappropriate variation found in the processes of the system. These include an understanding of the differences between enumerative and analytic techniques, the ability to measure random variation, the ability to identify "common" causes (also known as random causes) as opposed to "special" causes of variation in the system, and an understanding that inordinate attention to "common" causes damages the system rather than improves it (this forms an objective definition of "tampering" within a system).

Commitment to quality requires that objective measures of process and output be recorded, substantive knowledge be identified, then improvements to the processes that make up the system be implemented. The Shewhart Cycle describes a proven methodology for the detection and implementation of changes to a system that will result in higher quality and lower costs.

QUALITY OF SERVICE (DELIVERY QUALITY)

Quality is defined in terms of the wants and needs of the customers that an organization serves. It is therefore critical that the organization understand the wants, needs, perceptions, and expectations of its customer groups. For the purposes of this presentation (and the proposed model), these factors are grouped under the heading of Quality of Service. A first critical step in understanding customer satisfaction and expectations is to clearly define those customers an organization serves. As noted above, the definition of customer extends well beyond the group that uses an organization's final product—but the same principles that allow an organization to successfully satisfy its traditional customers can also be profitably applied to almost any other group with which the organization works.

For example, a hospital serves not only patients but patient families, physicians, health care financiers, and suppliers. A physician serves not only not only patients but other physicians and the hospital. A hospital department serves not only patients and physicians, but other departments within the hospital.

The hospital administration attempts to serve all groups associated with the hospital. In the past, some organizations have attempted to assess customer needs (as broadly defined above) by examining complaints that are brought to the organization. While this method has value in addressing the needs of individual customers (and of averting malpractice suits), it is seriously flawed as a means Of understanding the reaction of an entire customer population to the organization's products and services.

Recent research has shown that many customers, though extremely dissatisfied, never complain—they simply never return to the organization and advise all of their associates to stay away too. Sole concentration on complaints does not detect those problems, great and small, that customers consistently judge not to be worth the effort of a complaint. The chief tools for understanding the concerns, needs, and expectations of a broad customer population are questionnaires and customer focus groups.

A number of health care delivery researchers have made considerable progress in designing survey instruments to measure customer satisfaction (with customer broadly defined, as above) and to devise measurement systems that track progress in these areas, rather than setting artificial numerical goals. Of particular note is the work done by Paul Bataldan, M.D., at HCA, Inc., and Don Berwick, M.D., of the Harvard Community Health Plan. Quality in any industry is based upon the principle of continual innovation and improvement. However, most major innovations have not taken place in response to stated customer needs—for example, no customer focus group told Alexander Graham Bell that what was really needed was a device for communicating over tong distances through the use of electrical signals. The principle of innovation suggests that an organization will Study its Customers to understand their needs, even though the customers do not recognize those needs themselves.

The goal is to develop innovations that exceed—not meet—a Customer's reasonable expectations. Finally, it should be noted that good Customer service requires two-way communications. Customers can have reasonable expectations only if they understand the product, its natural limitations, and the proper way to use it.

VALUE OF CARE (CONTENT QUALITY)

While patients or other external customers determine expectations for the quality of delivery of medical care services, the medical content of care that is provided is still almost exclusively the province of the medical profession itself. This section therefore concerns itself with the quality of the content of medical care, as determined by health care professionals.

Value, as defined above, represents the combination of the quality of the medical care content that is delivered and the price (in terms of resources consumed) at which it is achieved. In order to treat a patient, a health care organization must have an infrastructure. It must have the necessary tools (which may be as simple as a stethoscope, or as complicated as a tertiary care hospital) and the necessary knowledge (as embodied in its professional medical staff) to intervene in disease processes with a positive result. Once the infrastructure is in place, a decision must be made to intervene (the diagnostic process) and a particular intervention (course of treatment) must be undertaken. The final result of this entire process is a health care outcome. Major areas that are considered include the following:

- *Establish the infrastructure.* A health care delivery organization must have the necessary physical plant and professional expertise to deliver high-quality care at a reasonable price. Hospitals have cooperated with the medical profession to establish processes that ensure professional quality, such as peer review, continuing medical education, and external standards. These efforts have largely been successful. While parts of the process may in some circumstances be improved (such as credentialing/privileging in some systems) the underlying principles of professional review are welt understood and usually welt applied. Humana's Allen Schaffer, M.D., has devised a computerized system that coordinates and manages the large number of external standards, propagated by a variety of external bodies, that a health care delivery system must satisfy. Issues regarding physical facilities for high value care are not well established. Improved analytic techniques are required to effectively address the acquisition of new technology (which may be very expensive and may at least partially duplicate existing, well established, capabilities), new procedures, and the siting of facilities within a hospital system to best serve a patient population.
- *Define indications for treatment.* A number of researchers have demonstrated a profound lack of clinical consensus on indications for treatment within a wide range of medical and surgical conditions. This lack of consensus is expressed as widely varying rates of utilization of particular procedures and treatments among the various regions of the country. Substantial improvements in both value of care and clinical outcome may be possible if better scientific knowledge regarding the clinical hypotheses that underlie a decision to institute treatment are available. Failures of diagnosis and clinical hypothesis usually result in quality waste.
- Evaluate cost versus output of competing treatment patterns. just

as there is a wide range of clinical opinions regarding indications for treatment, there is also a wide range of practice patterns once a decision to treat has been made. This has been shown by a number of studies regarding patterns of care, including the IHC QUE studies. As with indications for treatment, improvements in this area could lead to substantial improvements in both the value of care delivered and the outputs that are achieved. Failure to establish efficient patterns of care results in low productivity.

- *Avoid/mitigate errors.* Research into human-computer interfaces has confirmed what most health care professionals have always recognized: Humans are inherently imperfect information processors. When dealing with large amounts of complicated data (as in a medical setting) human errors and oversights will certainly occur, regardless of the level of expertise or attention given by the humans involved. Recognizing this inherent human deficiency, it is possible to build systems to crosscheck and verify decisions. These systems not only can prevent errors but also can lessen the impact of errors when they do occur. The focus should be on process, not just output, so that errors can be corrected before permanent harm results. Whether they are associated with failures in decisions to treat (diagnosis, evaluation of clinical hypotheses) or patterns of care (manner of intervention), treatment errors represent quality waste in its most straightforward form.
- *Improve the underlying medical science.* Medical science represents the product in which health care delivery organizations deal. Improvements in basic clinical knowledge allow health care professionals to improve the outcomes they can achieve and to reduce the costs necessary to reach a particular outcome. Some new treatments from which patients would benefit are available only in the research setting. Finally, an active programme of clinical research tends to attract the best physicians and ensures that they remain at the pinnacle of their profession. Ultimately, all of these factors serve to improve the value of care that a health care organization can deliver. Clinical research is equivalent to research and development in other industries.
- *Improve the delivery process.* Health care delivery research directly addresses the primary activity in which a health care system is engaged. Improvements in this process are critical factors for achieving and maintaining quality. Hospitals and other health care organizations have as much responsibility to improve the efficiency of their operations as physicians do to deliver only the highest quality medical care.

- Screen health care providers (physicians and hospitals) in terms of the outputs and outcomes they achieve. Case-adjusted analysis of outputs is a screening tool that can be used to detect potential deficiencies within a hospital or within a practice style. As a screening tool, these measures cannot prove that true deficiencies exist or locate them precisely within an organization. However, they can serve a very useful function in directing attention and further study to areas in which positive change might possibly be accomplished. The principle of continual improvement suggests that analysis of outputs should be extended to include the processes that result in a particular output. As clinical screening tools, these measures may be evaluated in terms of specificity and sensitivity, as with any other clinical screening test.

❒

Chapter - 3

Features of Health Planning

Since the Second World War, governments in Western industrialised countries have engaged in the planning of health services (Rodwin 1984). Health planning institutions and approaches have varied, but they have shared a common range of concerns. These include:

- How should health needs be assessed and met?
- How should a health system be organised and financed?
- What is the appropriate role and scale of hospitals? and
- What are the appropriate responsibilities for public health programmes?

Over the years the focus of health planning effort has changed. Health planning has evolved from the post-war expansionary phase to issues of cost containment and now to a concern with accountability and health outcomes. The early successes of creating a 'medical–industrial complex' have led, ironically, to a need to critically examine issues of effectiveness, efficiency and equity.

This chapter introduces the main theoretical issues and debates pertaining to planning in general and health planning specifically. It describes the different ways in which planning is conceived and practised. Definitions of key terms are provided. The fundamental dilemma of planning — whether to plan for health services or to plan for health improvement — is also raised.

WHAT IS PLANNING?

Planning can be thought of in numerous ways and is applicable to numerous activities. Most people try to arrange ahead many of the events of life. Budget planning is concerned with the allocation of limited and finite financial resources. Town planning is concerned with the control of influence on the future pattern of urban development and urban services. Most countries— at the national, state or local levels — engage in national security planning, economic planning, social planning, environmental planning and regional development planning. Dictionaries typically define the verb 'to plan' as meaning 'to arrange the parts of', 'to realise the achievement of' or 'to intend'. In the colloquial sense, then, 'planning' is concerned with deliberately achieving some objective by assembling actions into some orderly sequence. Green suggests that planning, as a separate identifiable activity in organisations, emerged from three strands of development. First, the rise of modern, complex industrial organisations in the late nineteenth century required decisions about the future to be taken in a considered and explicit manner.

Second, the Russian Revolution of 1917 led to the attempt to build an economy based on nationally determined plans and, hence, to the need for formal state planning (and planning bureaucracies). Third, the shortages experienced during the Second World War led to centralised controls in many Western countries.In Western industrialised democracies, planning as a generic activity and as a profession is commonly identified as emerging in the twentieth century, particularly after the Great Depression of the 1930s. Planning evolved as an attempt to mitigate the negative consequences of a laissez-faire market economy that was characterised by unrestrained pursuit of self-interest by individuals and corporations. The idea was for the state to intervene in markets through planning instruments in order to protect the collective interest. Public planning has thus had a long association with the notion of the welfare state and it has often been seen to be in conflict with private interests.Definitions of planning often reflect a tension between the technical tasks undertaken by the profession and the end objectives to be achieved by the tasks. In a generic and technical sense, planning can be conceived of as:

- 'the process of preparing a set of decisions for action in the future, directed at achieving goals by preferable means'; or
- 'making current decisions in the light of their future effects'. However, ways of thinking about planning have evolved with changes in society and the economy. In the 1940s, planning was concerned to set up the desired future end state in detail (that is, blueprint), but by the 1960s planning concentrated on the objectives of the plan and ways of obtaining them or systems planning. Hall suggests that, in the 1970s, planning became more heterogeneous and diffuse and it could be characterised as continuous participation in conflict. Friedmann would emphasise that planning, as the application of technical reasoning to specific

problems and leading to action or policy intervention, occurs in a social and political context.

Mainstream planners typically work for the state, although increasing numbers also work within civil society. The planning profession has historically seen the discipline as 'basically a methodology, a set of procedures applicable to a variety of activities aimed at achieving selected goals by the systematic application of resources in programmed quantities and time sequences designed to alter the projected trends and redirect them towards established objectives'. Such a perspective emphasises the technical and rational aspects of planning. Taylor and Reinke expand on this perspective when they agree that 'effective planning requires stepwise application of selected multidisciplinary methods and procedures to designated programmes and projects within specified time frames'. They add that 'planning is not simply a technical exercise; it is an ongoing process of learning, adapting to change and educating'.

As planners move into positions of facilitating change, the traditional model of rational planning is inserted into, if not transformed by, political practice. The values inherent in planning are made explicit by Blum. Planning, he says, 'is devoted to directing and attaining social changes of a specific and desired nature' and is the 'preferred means of achieving deliberate change'. Friedmann also sees planning practice as linking scientific and technical knowledge to processes of societal guidance, if not social transformation. In the 'societal guidance' model, planning is articulated through the state and is concerned with systematic change, while the political practice of system transformation becomes the focus on planning practice concerned with social transformation.

Parston suggests that planning is both an occupation and an idea. As an occupation, planning is work, a job. As an idea, planning is 'a process which is undertaken to meet some desired objective or to fulfil some purpose'. He argues they are inseparable. Forester also sees an activist role for the planner, in that planners are not only involved in problem solving; they are also concerned with problem finding or the mobilisation of attention to issues of concern.

As an activity that all organisations carry out with a greater or lesser degree of explicitness, planning involves making choices. When carried out by the public sector, planning is often conceived of as an intervention in the free market. In theory, the market allows equilibrium to be established between supply and demand as resources move in response to price signals. State intervention is limited and 'non-market goods' are produced in a complementary public sector. Classical economists see the market as the most efficient means of operating an economy. However, certain key conditions have to be met. These include good knowledge by the purchaser (or consumer) of the goods or services on offer, buyers and suppliers operating independently and the market operating independently to the extent that a purchase by one consumer does not necessarily affect the decision by another to purchase.

Planning, as an instrument of state intervention, has been justified on a number of grounds since the second half of the twentieth century. Milton Friedman, an economist who champions the free market, supports state intervention in the presence of natural monopolies and externalities. The liberal perspective suggests that state intervention is justified in order to correct market failure, to redistribute income and to manipulate fiscal and monetary policies in order to affect aggregate demand. Structuralist critiques of the state suggest that the contradictory need to maintain the conditions for capital accumulation and to raise revenue to meet its own obligation creates the need to convey an image of pursuing common and general interests of society as a whole, allowing access to power and responding to justified demands.

Planning has also been more recently criticised for its utilitarianism. Modern statecraft has been described as 'devoted to rationalising and standardising ... a social hieroglyph into a legible and administratively more convenient format'. State planning schemes can be seen as a means of social engineering, greater regimentation of communities and daily lives and enhanced state capacity.

Different conceptions of the role of the state will drive views on the nature and extent of state intervention required. For the health sector, views on the need for and the nature of, state intervention depend on whether the state is seen as regulator, service provider, financier or policy formulator for the health sector. In relation to health planning as a form of state intervention, the promarket position argues that health planning is likely to increase administrative controls and reduce professional autonomy and consumer choice. Health services delivery systems based on a professional model or a competitive free enterprise model would be favoured. The radical critique, in contrast, would see health as a right rather than a commodity and would prefer distribution of health resources on the basis of need. A model that requires central planning and regionalisation of health resources, such as the National Health Service in England prior to the Thatcher reforms, would be favoured. A mid-way position, represented by liberals, would accept a mixed system of public and private service provision and financing and focus state intervention on criteria such as accountability, rationality and equity.

Irrespective of their ideological positions, all governments ultimately need to make allocative decisions. Given that pure markets do not exist in the Australian context and that public sector financing and provision are dominant features, the setting of health care priorities is largely determined through health planning. The question, then, is not whether health care should be planned, but what to plan, by whom, how and when.

PLANNING TRADITIONS

Friedmann classifies the intellectual traditions of planning theory according to their political ideology as well as the intended use of knowledge.

The 'policy analysis' tradition derives from organisational theory, particularly how large organisations might improve their ability to make rational decisions. It is a rational–technical approach which builds on public administration, systems analysis and welfare and social choice theory and offers no distinctive philosophical position. The 'social reform' tradition is concerned with institutionalising planning practice and making action by the state more effective. Planners within this tradition tend to advocate a strong role for the state, which has both mediating and authoritative functions. Building on institutional economics and political sociology, they are interested in planning instruments and technical tools that help to manage the economy in the public interest.

The 'social learning' tradition is derived from organisational development approaches and focuses on the relationship between theory and practice. Rather than treating scientific knowledge as a set of building blocks for the reconstruction of society, planning is viewed as an ongoing dialectical process in which the main emphasis is on new practical undertakings.

Table. Intellectual traditions of Planning Theory

	Political ideology	
Knowledge to action	Conservative	Radical
In societal guidance	Policy analysis	Social reform
In social transformation	Social learning	Social mobilisation

The 'social mobilisation' tradition departs from all others by asserting the primacy of direct collective action from the grassroots (that is, the community). It is an ideology of the dispossessed, is concerned with social solidarity and aims to change the status quo. All of these traditions can be found in the brief history of health planning in Australia and they continue to co-exist. The Australian health care system has historically been characterised as a publicly planned and regulated system of supply. Even in the Australian private sector, risks are pooled through insurance arrangements and both private health care and insurance are heavily subsidised. Rational-technical planning models have been a feature of decision making about resource allocation in the health system for several decades.

At the same time, the Australian approach reflects strong cultural values about health care: that access should be determined by clinical need and not by the ability to pay; that people have a right to health care when they need it; and that health care is a key responsibility of government. Within this cultural context there have been significant shifts in policy, including a move away from institutional health care to community-based health services. Such policy debates and the ensuing processes of change often put planners within the social transformation mode. Green argues that the track record of planning internationally is often not good, as plans often fail either to be implemented or to respond to the real needs of the community. He suggests that failures arise due to:

- An emphasis on the formal process of planning, leading to it becoming a bureaucratic function or an end in itself;
- Technical failure to analyse needs appropriately or to estimate resources accurately;
- Imposition of plans from the centre in a top-down fashion, without involvement of providers and communities; and/or
- Isolation from other decision-making processes (such as budgets or human resources management).

The lessons are equally relevant to Australia and other countries — planning efforts will fail if planning is constructed as a narrow notion of apparently rational procedures being applied by a small group of technocrats who are oblivious to the broader political factors. Planning involves choices and change and, as such, will always have its opponents. Planning is neither ideology nor all powerful, but it does exist and have its effects. Understanding power structures and historical constraints, alongside the technical analysis and recognition of opportunities for action, is central to successful planning.

MODELS OF THE PLANNING PROCESS

Early planning thought is dominated by the comprehensive rational model. In this model the set of procedures essentially consists of:

- Goal setting, through identification of problems to be solved, needs to be met, opportunities to be seized and aspirations of stakeholders to be met.
- Plan formulation, through systematic analysis of alternatives, setting of criteria to choose amongst the options and examination of consequences of proposed actions.

- Plan implementation, through deploying a range of actions such as budgets, project schedules and regulatory measures.
- Monitoring and feedback, through reviewing achievements and updating the information, thus maintaining the currency of the plan. Such understanding of the planning process implies a systems view and a systems approach. The strength of this comprehensive, rational approach is that it is analytical, information-based and allows system design to be a central concern. It also allows for the introduction of normative thinking and valuation into planning. It is a set of technocratic or analytical processes that can be applied to a range of political and social contexts. The outcomes of the planning process reflect the definition of the planning problem, the information used for planning, the governance arrangements for the planning process and the extent to which the planning process is subject to public scrutiny.

The difficulties associated with this model — recognised over time — include the fact that planners seldom start with a blank slate and often do not have access to full information. The comprehensive rational planning model essentially conceives of planning as a technical and top-down activity led by expert planners. In reality, however, planning activities tend to be iterative with various activities occurring in parallel, rather than a chronologically ordered cycle of events. Furthermore, many problems require political rather than technical solutions. Non-etheless, the essential planning skills needed to cope with complex and changing environments can still be built upon the foundation of rational planning.

An alternative approach is the mixed scanning model advocated by Etzioni. Rather than considering comprehensively the alternatives for action, mixed scanning focuses only on selected areas of interest. Once the priority areas are chosen, the analytical process hones in on the marginal changes that are possible. This model is more pragmatic than the rational comprehensive model, insofar as it is a less costly process in terms of time and information resources. The analytical process is otherwise comparable. The critique of the rational planning model rests primarily in the political nature of planning. A third and distinct model is incrementalism, or what Lindblom terms 'muddling through'. The planning process is neither cyclical nor iterative, as the model is simply one of moving from the present position to the desired objectives by acting on a series of political windows of opportunity. The essence of this model is a series of disjointed steps, in contrast with the process of pure rationalism. Its emphasis on the political dimensions more accurately reflects the real world. It is also more flexible and allows for a faster response to changing environments.

However, incrementalism may serve to institutionalise existing power relations rather than encourage change, or it may lead to a lack of direction.

LEVELS OF PLANNING

Whether the model is comprehensive rationalism or mixed scanning, the analytical, problem-solving process outlined above can be applied to different levels of planning. These different levels are relevant across different fields of planning, be it health services, organisational development, urban affairs or military engagement.Dever outlines three levels of planning:

- Policy planning, which deals with what ought to be done, is the most conceptual and important in establishing system design. Planning at this level is normative and oriented towards future goals. There is also emphasis on design, on what should be rather than what is.
- Strategic planning, which deals with what can be done, is concerned with possible activities, implications for system structures and effectiveness and creation of instruments for action. The emphasis is on analysis (of need, of systems and institutions, or of stakeholders) which can lead to defining means to achieve desired goals.
- Operational planning, which deals with what will be done, is the most concrete. The focus is on specific activities to be undertaken and the resources required for implementation. The final outcome is an operational or implementation plan.

Friedmann places the levels of planning within a political and bureaucratic context. At the higher level of bureaucratic practice, planning may be focused on societal guidance and covers activities concerned with system maintenance and change. It is usually a top-down management of public affairs and incorporates policy planning and strategic planning as outlined above. The next level of bureaucratic practice is administrative planning. This involves both management of programme routines and developing processes for institutional change. It is comparable to operational planning above.

STYLES OF PLANNING

Planning at the macro level can be seen as synonymous with policy making. Planning becomes a process of strategy formulation with concerns focused on power in political systems, consensus versus conflict views of how society functions and questions about issues such as the role of government, the media, interest groups, political parties and global politics.A more instrumentalist perspective tends to inform planning as strategy development at the organisational level. Mintzberg sees strategy development in organisations as occurring in one of three ways:

- Leader-driven strategy, where the strong leader determines strategy.
- Adaptive strategy, where small (often disjointed) reactive steps are taken to resolve problems/issues (incrementalism).
- Formal planning (rationalism), where analysis is used to develop explicit strategies.

Some organisations rely on the visions and strategies of a single charismatic or powerful leader who may derive their power from expertise, position, shared values or ideas, or coercion. Such a top-down approach is likely to discourage others from being innovative and creative. Further, it does not recognise the increased effectiveness associated with collaboration with communities and stakeholders.

In contrast, adaptive or power–behavioural approaches rely on negotiation, bargaining and the importance of coalitions. This approach recognises that multiple goals can co-exist in organisations and that there is a need to constantly reflect, plan and amend strategies. Incrementalism can be a useful perspective as it provides for organisational plurality, supports an analysis of organisational power and questions whose interests will be served through a particular strategy. But it may also lead to 'muddling through' without direction.

Formal planning can provide a set of concepts, directions and procedures to help people to think and act strategically, with a view to developing a comprehensive short- and long-term agenda. Formal processes can potentially provide an organised approach to developing innovative ideas and for involving people at all levels. A plan, however, is best seen as just one building block in a series of events that determine macro-level strategy (Quinn 1991). Moreover, there is a wide variety of values and approaches to formal planning which may be more or less participatory, planned or impulse-driven, top- down or bottom-up, implicit or explicit, focused on the past or on the future, or concerned with both.

Macro-level strategic planning often involves a mixture of formal planning, incrementalist (power–political) processes and management techniques, depending on the issue and context. There may even be times when openness to new ideas, information and approaches and a strong commitment to a particular issue or goal are more important than a brilliant strategic analysis. Hall et al. suggest that when an issue has high legitimacy, feasibility and support, it is likely to become an agenda item.Insofar as planning is an activity concerned with effecting change, the planner is not a neutral technocrat. Benveniste suggests two essential approaches to planning in terms of how the planner defines his/her role:

- Advocacy planning, where planning is a means of redressing the imbalances between different groups with different power and the role of the planner is to take an active role in facilitating change.
- Apolitical planning, where planning is the use of technical knowledge to achieve political or managerial compromise.

In the classification offered by Friedmann, 'apolitical planning' is comparable to 'allocative planning', which is concerned with distribution of scare resources among competing claimants or uses. 'Advocacy planning', however, is sub-divided into 'institutional planning' and 'radical planning', with the former oriented towards facilitating institutional change and the latter attempting to draw on organised citizen power to promote social transformation. The former can also be conceived of as adopting a pluralist approach involving negotiations with key stakeholders and communities to reach an equilibrium or consensus. The latter, on the other hand, may adopt a structuralist analysis and be based on collaboration between planners and communities in order to confront and address the determinants of inequity. Sandercock offers a typology of planning approaches based on the evolution of urban planning models. These include:

- The rational comprehensive model, where the planner is indisputably the expert.
- The advocacy planning model, where the planner represents the interests of the disadvantaged (though leaving intact the workings of plural democracy).
- The radical political economy model, where planning is an instrument of the capitalist state and the planner's role is as the revealer of contradictions and an agent of social innovation.
- The equity planning model, where the planning effort consciously seeks to redistribute power, resources or participation.
- The social learning and communicative action model, which acknowledges the value of local and experiential knowledge.
- The radical or emancipatory planning model, where the planner's allegiance is to the community rather than the state and his/her role is to work for social transformation through community-based organisations.

In examining the evolution of planning practice, Sandercock suggests some new pillars for post-modern planning:

- Greater and explicit reliance on practical wisdom;
- People-centred, as opposed to focusing on the planning document;
- Need to access multiple ways of knowing (for example, community experiences);
- Greater emphasis on community empowerment; and
- Recognition of the existence of multiple publics and developing multicultural literacy.

She stresses different sources of information and evidence for planning, with the keys being: knowledge through dialogue; knowledge from experience; learning from local knowledge; learning to read symbolic and non-verbal evidence; learning through contemplative or appreciative knowledge; and learning by doing, or action planning.

The inherently value-laden nature of planning thus raises some critical questions about who should be involved in the planning process, how they should be involved and when they should be involved. The answers to these questions are often informed by an understanding of why a planning process is being undertaken. It can be asked:

- Is planning an aid or replacement to political decision making?
- Is planning a means of improving social justice?
- Is planning a means of getting some focus on the future?
- Is planning a gentle, persuasive route to turn ideas into action?
- Is planning a method for shared decision making?
- Is planning a means of improving the quality of effort applied to problem solving?
- Is planning a means of control?

Clarity about the answers to the above questions will result in different ways to resolve the issues which frequently occur in 'doing' planning, such as:

- What should be the process for developing a plan?
- Who should write the plan (for example, consultants, planners or managers)?
- What are the merits of a centralised versus decentralised approach?
- Who should be involved in the planning activities (for example, managers or consumers)?

- What should be the governance arrangement for the planning process?
- What are the merits of group consultation versus individual consultation?

Some of these questions may appear to be purely technical, yet most embody notions about the distribution of power, the winners and losers in any changes to the status quo and the legitimacy of the planning exercise as perceived by the stakeholders.

PARTICULAR FEATURES OF HEALTH PLANNING

The particular features that distinguish health planning from other forms of planning relate to the peculiarity of the health system. Palmer and Short suggest that the distinctiveness of health policy results from three broad defining factors:

- The unique role of the medical profession;
- The complexity of health care; and
- The nature of community expectations and values associated with health.

Some see that health care is distinguished by its hierarchical nature and by the dominance of the medical profession. Medical dominance is seen as being achieved through professionalism (freedom from scrutiny), authority over other health workers and professionals and by shaping social beliefs and understandings about health. Furthermore, the orientation towards curative care, including resource allocation to this area, is reinforced by the nature of the medical profession. Shortell and Kaluzney identify a number of operational features that distinguish health care organisations. While they recognise that many other organisations may possess one or more of these features, health care organisations will display a combination of these factors. Amongst these are:

- Definition and measurement of output is difficult.
- Work is variable and complex.
- Work is likely to be emergency work.
- There is little capacity for error.
- Activities require considerable coordination amongst a range of professional groups.
- Work is highly specialised.
- Workers are highly professionalised with strong allegiances to their profession.

- There is little control over doctors, yet they generate the costs.
- Dual lines of authority often operate.

Hospitals, of all health service organisations, may be particularly impervious to changes in the external environment. As 'closed systems', hospitals have what Taylor described as the hospital's 'cult of efficiency': long-established work patterns, routines, roles and power relations. The hierarchy is maintained with tight scheduling, numerous rules and regulations and control mechanisms.

The rigidity, control, tight scheduling and official rules and regulations in health service institutions have long been critiqued. Health service agreements, awards, commitments and understandings also serve to mitigate against organisational change. The bureaucratic culture is determined by the accumulation of the decisions of clinicians.

In more recent times, the traditional power base of doctors may have been partly eroded in the face of health care reform, managerialism, the strengthening power base of other professions in the health field (including economists, planners, nurses, lawyers and alternative medicine), unremitting cost control and the growth of active consumer interest groups. Organisational boundaries are also being blurred with horizontal integration and collaboration between hospitals and community-based health services and between the private and public sectors. Networks of services are increasingly becoming more useful descriptions of the health system.

The complexity of promoting health in the face of increasing societal inequity and environmental degradation is challenging health professionals to work in different ways.Health planning has also been challenged by the rapid pace of change. Public sector reforms, including the introduction of purchaser–provider split models, initially raised questions about whether there is a role for state planning. Experience with formula-based output payments, however, still suggests that the state health authority has to plan for the volume and types of services to be purchased. More recently, purchasers have learned that their planning needs to be at a finer level, since the need for health services is a more specific concept than the need for health.The particular features of the health system described above have several implications.

One is the relationship between health management, health planning and clinical practice. Should health planning be an integral component of health management? Should health planning be the bridge between clinical practice, health management and the political process? Should health planning be the process by which clinical knowledge is channelled to drive health system reform? Another important issue is the relationship between health planning and health financing and accounting. Should health planners be advocates for health and for patients? Should health planners be technicians involved in the distribution of finite health dollars? Should health planners be the decision makers who decide what to purchase in a purchaser–provider relationship? In practice, all of these roles are present in health planning to a greater or lesser extent. Health planning is thus practised in an environment where technical and bureaucratic traditions exist simultaneously with complexity and change on both technological and social dimensions.

MODELS OF HEALTH PLANNING

Health planning is essentially concerned with improving health and with improving health services delivery or system performance. These two aims, however, require somewhat different approaches to planning. A planning effort concerned with improving population health (also called population- based planning) usually employs the following iterative process:

- Select health issue(s) of concern.
- Identify risks.
- Evaluate population risk levels (at present and in future).
- Select programmes to eliminate or reduce risks.
- Compare needed programmes with existing programmes.
- Adjust resources.
- Evaluate.

A planning exercise focused on improving health services delivery (also known as institution-based or resource-based planning) is also iterative and may use similar logic but has different starting points. The general model is:

- Select health service(s) of concern.
- Determine current demand.
- Forecast potential demand.
- Compare forecast with present resource capacity.
- Adjust resources.
- Evaluate.

Despite comparable logic, there are significant differences between the two models in orientation and methodological requirements. The population-based planning model establishes resource requirements based upon assessment of the risk levels and the health status of a given population. As such, it incorporates a broader understanding of the determinants of health, particularly the social and environmental factors influencing health outcomes. Its tendency is to focus on preventive programmes and reorientate the health care system towards primary health care. It also gives recognition to the need for intersectoral collaboration and for community action in achieving health status improvement. Its main problems rest with gaining an accurate assessment of health status and risk levels and testing the capacity of the health sector to influence broader determinants of health.

The resource-based planning model can be applied to a service or a facility. It is largely an attempt to match supply with demand and its implementation is concerned with adjustments within the existing delivery system, most commonly with rationalisation of existing resources. This form of health planning is the dominant approach.

At a broader level, the differences in population-based and resource-based planning models also reflect different political interests. The resource-based approach is largely concerned with institutional growth and development and serves the dominant interests of the institutional sector. In the health sphere, the dominant institution is the hospital and the dominant interest it serves is the medical profession. The population-based approach, on the other hand, is concerned (by definition) with community and societal interests. It requires the planner (and the planning body) to address the needs of the population as the central issue in the planning process and, as such, to become an advocate for community interests.

The history of health planning is characterised by movement from facilitybased planning to a focus on health outcomes. This reflects a number of important trends. First, there has been a shift in health policy, from expansion of hospital facilities to the need to rationalise resources, through to a concern for the health return on the investment. Second, this shift in orientation itself has reflected the contest in policy space between dominant professional interests and community and consumer interests, supported by 'corporate rationalisers'. Third, there has been a shift from relegating planning to a technical analytical function, to becoming an integral part of management if not an approach to management. It can be expected, then, that the judicious combination of resource-based planning and population-based planning will be the direction for future development.

Health planning operates in a complex and changing environment. Planning can be highly technical or solely political. It can be done to help with 'muddling through' of daily decision making or with a radical envisioning of the future system. The essential problem faced by health planners is as follows. While there is general agreement among policy makers and the community that all people should enjoy good health and have access to health care, planners are not and have not been, able to specify what constitutes an optimal system of health and related services for keeping the population healthy. The challenge is not solely in the technical design of a health system. Insofar as a health system reflects societal norms and expectations as well as the resources available, planning is a political process and requires a multitude of tools for implementation. The planning predicament, then, embodies the tasks associated with leveraging support for action.

CORE HEALTH PLANNING PRINCIPLES

There are a number of planning parameters which are commonly used and essentially form the 'language' of health planning. The core health planning principles include equity, accessibility, efficiency, quality and effectiveness. Each is discussed in turn.

EQUITY

Equity in health planning is often defined as equity of access, which means that an individual will receive an equal opportunity to receive health care, irrespective of personal characteristics such as income, race, gender or place of residence. Equity may be assessed through consideration of the definition of the target group, the methods for promoting access and analysis of the geographical or locational equity.

An important alternative concept is equity of outcome, which refers to the fairness of the outcomes from a particular health care intervention or service. This approach to equity takes into account the range of sociological, economic and other factors that may mitigate against a fair distribution of health chances. Equity of outcome implies the need for redistribution such that new or additional resources are targeted to redress inequity.

ACCESSIBILITY

Access is the capacity or potential to obtain a service or benefit. Access incorporates notions of geographical access, physical/architectural access, cultural/ linguistic access, service acceptability and affordability. Service accessibility may refer to several things: geographical accessibility (for example, travel time to the service, or transport routes); cultural accessibility (for example, availability of interpreters for non-English-speaking background (NESB) immigrants, Aboriginal health workers, or the appropriateness of the environment for young people); physical accessibility (for example, ramps for disabled people or people with prams); service availability (for example, waiting times, opening hours, access for people working and so on); or financial access (that is, whether the cost of a service constitutes a barrier).

EFFICIENCY

Efficiency focuses on the maximisation of total benefits from the use of a given amount of resources. Technical efficiency, or productive efficiency, refers to maximising service or strategy outputs by using minimal inputs. In some social services, measures of efficiency are defined as being synonymous with costeffectiveness in that they relate outcome to input (such as the cost of obtaining one extra year of life). In this book, efficiency will be related to service outputs, not to outcomes.

The efficiency of a particular service or strategy can be assessed or planned for in a number of ways. One approach is to compare the service or strategy to other similar services/strategies on the basis of agreed outputs. It may be important that these output indicators be adjusted to reflect casemix, where such information is available.

Allocative efficiency is concerned with maximising the health and welfare of the community through ensuring an appropriate distribution of benefits. This is particularly important in considering the balance of investment between inpatient and community-based services, between preventive and curative services and between ongoing professional care and the self-help and support services provided by lay volunteers.

Dynamic efficiency is concerned with adaptability of the system over time. It is an economic concept that has yet to come to the fore in the health arena, but it can be expected to assume greater prominence as issues of sustainability attract greater attention.

QUALITY

Quality measures the degree to which a health care professional or service conforms to pre-set standards. Quality measures may include process measures (that is, the activities undertaken as a part of the service) or outcome measures (that is, the result). Ideally, both process and outcome measures would be used.

Information on the quality of processes can be obtained through analysing selected performance measurements (for example, casemix adjusted measures of complication errors, medication errors, transfers to higher levels of care, readmission rates, customer satisfaction, employee surveys, timeliness, waste and defects) or by generating information on a particular issue (for example, the proportion of people with acute myocardial infarction who receive streptokinase treatment within an hour of arriving at hospital).

FFECTIVENESS/OUTCOMES

Effectiveness is the level of benefit when a service is rendered under ordinary circumstances by average practitioners for typical patients. This is distinct from the concept of efficacy (the level of benefit expected when health services are applied under ideal conditions). A health outcome is a change in the health of individuals or a group of people or populations that can be attributed wholly or partially to a health intervention or a series of interventions. The key issue is how to identify the best indicators or measures of benefit or health gain. Health gain indicators, or 'outcome measures', should be directly relevant both to the health needs and to the health intervention. For instance, the percentage of the infant population immunised is a relevant indicator for an immunisation campaign. When the immunisation level can be attributed to the intervention (in this case, the immunisation campaign), it can constitute a 'health outcome'. When it cannot be attributed to the intervention, the percentage immunised is a 'health status' measure and not a 'health outcome' measure.

A service should ideally collect and analyse its own data on the outcomes of its interventions. If the service is provided as part of a broader treatment/ care stream (for example, physiotherapy post-orthopaedic surgery), it is difficult to undertake outcome evaluation as outcome evaluation is best undertaken across a whole service intervention. Services should identify whether the target group is an individual or a population. Consumers/ communities should ideally be involved in deciding the value of the outcomes of the service/intervention. There are often difficulties in obtaining valid information about outcomes in ordinary service settings, due to differences in consumers/target groups/communities and the multiple factors that may influence outcomes.

As reflected by the core principles of health planning, most of the planner's work is concerned with the efficient and effective delivery of health care services. Does health planning actually make a difference to health status or the level of health experienced by individuals and communities? The answer to this question is complicated by differing understandings of what health is and what health planners do.

DEFINITIONS OF HEALTH

There are many definitions of health. Health can be defined by its presence or its absence and it can have individual or societal parameters. In 1946 the World Health Organisation (WHO) defined health as 'a state of complete physical, mental and social well-being and not merely the absence of disease or infirmity' (WHO 1946). In this definition, health is defined as a positive experience rather than the absence of sickness and as a social rather than a solely individual phenomenon. Critics argue that it defines health as 'perfect health', a concept which is unable to be measured or obtained and is always future-oriented.

Definitions of health and what health planners do, however, vary according to the frames of reference used. Doctors, administrators and consumers may view health differently and therefore have different views on how health needs should be met, what health services are needed and how they should be delivered. Major health frames of references include biological/ biomedical, clinical health sciences, population health, ecological public health, social health and everyday life. Planners typically focus on population issues, morbidity and demography.

DETERMINANTS OF HEALTH

The causes of illness are complex and the social, cultural and environmental impacts on health are now well documented. The determinants of health interact in complex ways, with diseases sharing common risk factors and risk factors clustered in socioeconomic groups.

Broad determinants of health may include socioeconomic structures, physical, human-made and ecological environments, health service access or quality, individual biology, cultural beliefs, personal behaviour and lifestyle choices. Specific determinants may include nutrition, infectious agents, trauma, congenital or inherited problems, the physical environment (sun, radiation, altitude), tobacco and alcohol consumption, age, gender, occupation, stress and social isolation. Epidemiological evidence increasingly points to the importance of social factors in explaining health status differences across populations.

Epidemiology is at the core of contemporary understanding of the distribution and causation of health and disease at the population level. Over the past 150 years, epidemiological concepts have undergone a number of shifts, from infectious disease epidemiology (based on germ theory) to the 'classic triad' (physical, genetic and environment causes), to the current interest in chronic diseases and multiple risk factors.

Contemporary public health approaches critique both the biomedical model and an 'illness-centred' focus on the physical risk factors of individuals and groups. The more comprehensive 'web of causation' takes biological and social factors and interventions into account and may span the genetic to the societal. The central concept in the web of causation is that many variables may be related to a single effect through direct and indirect causes. The main evidence for determinants of health comes from the prevalence of disease differences between different population sub-groups. The available data about the distribution of determinants are often poor, however and this makes planning for health (with any sophistication) difficult.

If the ultimate goal of health planning activities is to impact positively on health status, then decisions have to be taken about which of the myriad of factors/determinants are priorities for action and what can be done about them. Certainly, it is not necessary (even were it possible) to understand causal mechanisms fully in order to undertake prevention. The knowledge of small components in the web of causation can significantly contribute to prevention or improved treatment/therapy. The Ottawa Charter suggests five core strategies for health improvement: building healthy public policy; creating supportive environments; strengthening community action; developing personal skills; and reorienting health services. The challenge in health planning is to act successfully on the social determinants of health.

HEALTH SERVICES AND THEIR IMPACT ON HEALTH STATUS

The importance of public health measures in improving health has long been recognised. The dramatic decline in mortality in the last 100 years has been widely attributed to the first public health revolution resulting in environmental improvements, including sanitation, nutrition, water supply, housing and education. These improvements led to significant overall declines in infectious diseases such as tuberculosis, typhus-typhoid, cholera, dysentery and diarrhoea, smallpox and scarlet fever. Medical and scientific advances such as the development of antibiotics, the development of the Salk and Sabin vaccines for poliomyelitis and developments in surgery contributed to reduced death rates in the 1950s; however, these only marginally improved mortality rates. The decline in population mortality in the last century has coincided with, rather than been caused by, the rise of modern medicine.

The impact of medical access on overall health status is likely to be less than the impact of improving working and living conditions. Current studies estimate that 60–80 per cent of current disease is preventable through social change. The Center for Disease Control in the United States attributed only 10 per cent of premature mortality to inadequate health care.

Despite the contention that medical interventions have a relatively marginal impact on the overall mortality levels of a community, medicine generally enjoys great community credence. Science and the scientific method is most frequently credited with having the explanations for illness and health and the 'curative' health system continues to consume the bulk of the health budget.

Nevertheless, whilst national mortality rates tend not to respond to increases in hospital and medical resources, medical care does contribute to the reduction of non-fatal diseases, disability, discomfort and distress.

Health services extend life through interventions such as immunisation, accident and trauma services and cancer treatments. Quality of life may also be improved through relief of pain, improved mobility (joint replacements) and effective treatment of many non-life-threatening conditions. The challenge for health planning is to ensure equitable access to costeffective health care while harnessing complementary strategies for health improvement.

PLANNING FOR EQUITY AND HEALTH

Equity or fairness in health has been defined as a 'focus on the distributional impact of health policies on different individuals and families'. Health inequality can be defined as differences in health status, whereas health inequity links differences in health to social injustice and implies unfairness and the need for amelioration. Equity in health, whilst often appearing in the rhetoric of plans or policies, is rarely adequately examined and is differentially understood and applied, despite being generally applauded as a planning goal.

There are (at least) three main approaches to equity in health: equity as the minimum standard equity of access; and equity of outcome.

EQUITY OF ACCESS AND EQUAL HEALTH CARE

Equity is achieved when an individual receives equal health care irrespective of personal characteristics such as income, race, gender or place of residence. This does not imply equal treatment in the sense of the same treatment. Rather, the treatment or care should be tailored to meet diverse individual needs and circumstances (for example, providing an interpreter for a patient who does not speak English). This approach has been the goal of much policy and planning in the last 30 years.

EQUITY OF OUTCOME

Equity is achieved when the outcomes from a health care intervention — regardless of whether it is intersectoral, prevention, treatment or palliation — are fairly distributed across population groups and individuals. Where the current distribution of outcomes is unfair, this approach provides for redistribution. Consistent with this view, a public health approach, for example, would define equity as 'affirmative action on any resource differentially distributed in the community — for example, housing, education, income and political power. It implies access to these resources by those with the least opportunities at present'.Key questions in health planning therefore include:

- Should plans focus solely on the health care sector, or is a broad-based multisectoral approach required?

- Should equity of outcome replace equity of access? As a corollary, should a goal be to simply maintain (but not improve) the current health standing of advantaged Australians whilst new resources are targeted to improve the health status of the most disadvantaged groups?

A BRIEF HISTORY OF HEALTH PLANNING

Health planning trends have followed the prevailing and shifting policy paradigms of the last 30 years. An initial focus on equity and access had shifted by the 1980s to a concern with equity and efficiency. By the 1990s/2000s the accelerated efficiency drive led to a concern about the quality and effectiveness of health interventions. Planning has evolved from an initial concern with developing much-needed data and information, through to developing normative planning standards which sought to define system and service inputs and then to a concern with outcomes, effectiveness and change management.

The changes in the paradigms have been complemented by ongoing tensions between community/public health services and traditional hospital and institutional approaches, between prevention and treatment, between the bureaucracy versus health providers and, inevitably and most recently, between market forces and planning. The dilemmas associated with developing a broader community-centred, consultative and ecological approach to health have also emerged.

This chapter provides an overview of health planning in Australia, concentrating on its evolution since the 1970s. Health planning practice has essentially developed in three streams. Hospital planning has focused on locational distribution and efficiency of service delivery. Community health services planning has been concerned with equity and population health need. The presence of more specialised planning practice — be it workforce or technology — has reflected policy demands. The planning skills of the health planner have increasingly moved into the corporate planning arena.

EARLY HISTORY OF HEALTH PLANNING

At the start of the twentieth century there was little other than basic population information on which to plan and there was considerable political interference in priority setting. Indeed, hospitals and health services were generally established for political gain, just prior to an election. Until the 1970s, special interest and advocacy groups (aside from medical and professional interest groups) were rare.

Hospitals were established with little detailed planning and without regard to related services. Bed numbers and roles were contrived by comparison with existing hospitals. In the major cities, hospitals were generally built in the inner city areas. In the rural areas, it was expected that each town should have its own hospital and that a town should be 'no more than a horse ride away' (fifteen minutes by motor vehicle). Irrespective of the size of their catchment population, rural towns generally had an acute hospital that also provided nursing home type services. Hospitals, at this time, were relatively inexpensive to operate and when budgets were overspent the government simply increased the budget. There was a political view that hospital costs had to be met and there was little pressure on health administrators or politicians to contain costs.

Up to the 1970s, public health issues were largely dominated by a biomedical approach. Mass immunisations and screening had been undertaken in the post-war period to eradicate or control diseases such as tuberculosis and polio. By the 1970s, awareness had developed about the problems associated with an 'affluent society': smoking, drinking, obesity and traffic accidents.

Prior to the 1970s, governments tended to respond to concerns about health care direction or decision making by establishing commissions of inquiry or special senate task forces, comprising medical experts and politicians who would identify key recommendations for future action. Whilst significant changes occurred in health services during these first seven decades of the last century, little formal planning was involved. Planning was effectively entwined with the political process.

COMPREHENSIVE HEALTH PLANNING DEVELOPS

A Division of Planning and Research and began to assess the equity of service provision in the state. This process highlighted the lack of health services in the west of Sydney in comparison to the inner city areas. The first comprehensive service plan was a plan for the rapidly growing south-west of Sydney, incorporating Campbelltown and Liverpool. This plan was revolutionary for its day in that it demonstrated the existing health service's locational inequities and also planned for the full range of services, including hospitals, community health, a new generalist community nurse service and mental health. A similar planning exercise was undertaken for the Mt Druitt area, where a polyclinic rather than a hospital was planned. By the late 1970s the unit had developed the first metropolitan-wide health service plan. Such plans required enormous technical effort, as there was little readily available data. With the incoming Whitlam government a reformist agenda was introduced at the national level, with the introduction of national health insurance and the Community Health Programme (CHP) as key features. Sidney Sax moved from New South Wales to the Commonwealth to head up the newly established Hospitals and Health Services Commission (HHSC) in 1973. This body developed policies concerning the supply and distribution of health services and established a national health service planning model. The model envisaged a network of services comprised of primary care, private specialist care, hospitals, nursing homes, hostels and rehabilitation and domiciliary care. Of central importance were the primary care teams.

The Commission also developed the first national normative planning standards for health service provision, which were particularly pertinent for the development of the CHP. Amongst these standards were that a community of 6000 people should have two to three general practitioners and two community nurses and that communities with 40 000 people should have a community health centre, with facilities and services to support the primary care teams. The impact of the CHP on health planning was far-reaching, extending beyond the Commonwealth in that it required the introduction of populationbased planning into the state-based health system.

In response to the Whitlam government's policy of augmenting and upgrading hospitals, the Commonwealth HHSC undertook a national study of the needs and distribution of Australian hospitals. The survey highlighted the inequitable distribution of hospital beds between inner city areas and newly developed outer areas in several states. The report found an oversupply of beds in rural areas. The study suggested that the number of beds per 1000 population in Australia (6.3 beds per 1000) was too high. It recommended that Commonwealth financial assistance should be based on assessed need (that is, policy), rather than being merely a per capita distribution. This effectively constituted the first comprehensive national plan for health care in Australia. However, as often occurs in health planning, the government preempted the report and announced capital grants for the development of Westmead Hospital in Sydney, Western Suburbs Geriatric Centre and Hospital in Melbourne and the Mt Gravatt Hospital in Brisbane.

DATA DEVELOPMENT BECOMES IMPORTANT

During the planning process the Commonwealth identified a 'serious shortage of the kind of information that is essential for the planning and evaluation of health services at all levels'. In 1973, the Commonwealth responded by providing a matched grant programme of $1.025 million a year. This comprised $500 000 to support the development of state-based health services planning and research, $500 000 to universities and colleges and $25000 for seminars on data collection, record systems, planning and evaluation. Specific research training programmes were included in later years. These funds were to be used by the states to develop their planning and research capacities. Until this time, health services planning and research outside New South Wales was poorly developed. It was hoped that biomedical researchers would be enticed into health service planning and teach research skills to bureaucrats involved in planning. The role envisaged for research was to study need, access to services, productivity, efficiency and cost control. The role envisaged for planning was one of providing research findings to health service administrators, with the view that providing such advice might facilitate more rational policy. These grants provided an impetus for the development of health planning as a profession and for the establishment of state and regional planning functions.

In the 1970s there was little planning data other than population statistics. Annual reports of health authorities were only able to report the states' bed capacity, the average length of stay and the daily average, the number of newborn babies and the numbers who attended outpatient services. The hospital billing system provided additional basic data sets, as did hospital surveys. There was, however, no health status or diagnosis information and no patient information. Therefore, for health planning to be taken seriously by health administrators and politicians, significant technical and research effort was required. Consequently, the development of planning tools, including information systems, became an important priority for most planning units. For example, in its annual report in 1977/78, the Commonwealth's proud boast was that it had developed its 'computer based information bank. It now contains demographic and statistical information on hospitals, nursing homes and other institutions ... inappropriate levels of services can thus be identified' (Commonwealth Department of Health).

The first Hospital Morbidity Data Collection was developed in the Riverina area of New South Wales in the early 1960s. The departmental officer representing the NSW Health Commission successfully argued the case for statewide hospital morbidity collection, health surveys and perinatal statistics on the basis that it was 'reprehensible that the state knew more about its sheep than its people!'. By 1977 the completion of hospital morbidity data became mandatory in New South Wales and by 1978 this requirement was extended to private hospitals. The general and psychiatric collections were integrated at this time. This provided a prototype for data on the health status of populations.

The data items included in the collection were demographic variables, diagnoses and operations. There was considerable negative reaction to the requirement to complete data returns from hospitals, as it was considered that this would take medical resources away from clinical care. There was also suspicion about how the data would be used. There was, at this time, no national agreement on definitions and approaches. The process of collecting and entering data was laborious. Data would arrive on paper and had to be transferred to punch cards. Data were all centrally processed by the Australian Bureau of Statistics.

The need for more uniform approaches to hospital capital works led to the establishment of a variety of planning bodies. In New South Wales, the Hospital Planning Advisory Council was established in 1973 to develop key capital planning parameters, undertake planning research and develop tools such as the 'hospital planning units' which provided capital planning standards relating to the size, location and general functionality of hospital and health services. In 1975 a Household Health and Welfare Survey was conducted in the Gosford–Wyong and Illawarra areas of New South Wales by the NSW Division of Planning and Research in conjunction with the Commonwealth Bureau of Statistics. The survey aimed to assess acute and chronic health problems and the health services used by the people. This became the pilot National Health Survey, which is now an important regular source of health status information.

Linking resource allocation issues to health planning was also recognised. In 1975, New South Wales developed a rudimentary 'resource allocation formula' based on the approach undertaken in Britain. Again, this formula provided a model for future population-based resource allocation exercises.

The 1970s witnessed significant new directions for health system development that began to require the advice of 'experts'. Planners were initially innovative researchers who had to 'order spreadsheets from central office by mail. They hand-drew column graphs and scatter charts and added up large numbers of hospital separations on pocket calculators to assess admission trends'.

With these beginnings, planning emerged as a technical support to the bureaucracy. Planners developed new data and information sources and began to develop normative planning standards which could define service and system inputs. Planners became experts in analysing hospital separation, mortality and demographic data as a means of assessing a community's health needs.

PRIORITY SETTING AS A PLANNING ROLE EMERGES

During the second half of the 1970s the economic environment began to change. In 1975 the incoming Liberal Fraser government questioned the efficiency of public hospitals and developed policies to force the states to establish cost control mechanisms. Health care costs had increased from about 5 per cent of GDP in 1963/64 to 7.7 per cent in 1975/76.

Planning remained in the service of decision makers, but the goal was to discourage hospital use. Bed planning ratios of four acute beds per 1000 people were established and in 1978 the Commonwealth–State cost-sharing agreement required that equal numbers of beds should be closed if new beds or services were to be opened.

The Fraser government instigated a range of cost control measures designed to regulate the expansion of hospital beds and services, the supply of practitioners, the development of community health and the consumer contribution to health care. The significant changes in the health policy environment meant that planning was not a means of developing comprehensive new services but a tool to assist in or to justify cost cutting. Planning became more integrated into management decision making.

PLANNING FOCUSES ON INCREASING HOSPITAL EFFICIENCY

In 1980 the Commission of Inquiry into the Efficiency and Administration of Hospitals reported that health information systems were inadequate and that hospital administration appeared to be inefficient. It recommended a reduction in the number of hospital beds per 1000 population and that states develop comprehensive health service plans which would outline the development of all components of the health system on a regional and statewide basis.

Increasing pressure on the hospital budget, leading to greater support for non-hospital care, resulted from several factors: reduced hospital revenues arising from Medicare changes in 1981; the introduction by the Commonwealth of the '35 day rule' which limited acute hospital coverage to 35 days; increasing hospital staffing costs associated with the 38-hour week; requirements for improved health and safety; quality control procedures; and the safeguarding of patients' rights to informed consent.

Hospital cost control measures implemented at this time concentrated mainly on instruments such as patient payments to deter use and budgetary controls. In the 1970s, hospital administrators who spent in excess of their budget would be regularly 'bailed out' by the central-leveladministration, but by the 1980s this had changed (that is, 'come in on budget or your job may be on the line'). There was increased productivity in public hospitals during this time.

Hospital productivity improvements arose from a decrease in length of stay, an increase in same day procedures (both due in large part to the development of less invasive surgical techniques and anaesthetics and improved diagnostic technologies), early and supported discharge for some types of care (especially ophthalmology and obstetrics) and an increase in non-inpatient or ambulatorycare as an alternative to admission (for example, home dialysis, community-basedpalliative care and diabetic management).

Information systems developed significantly. Planners and managers were able to question the variability between different hospitals and within a hospital: the costs of individual patient care; average length of stay; number of admissions; waiting times; numbers of operations; admissions through emergency departments and so on. However, the hospitals invariably claimed that such variability was due to variations in the age and complexity of the patient mix.

At this time, information tools which had the capability for controlling for patient mix were being developed in the United States. By the mid-1980s the Victorian Health Department and the South Australian Health Commission initiated studies into the usage of the US Diagnosis Related Group (DRG) classification as an approach to allocating funds to hospitals. By the end of the 1980s the Commonwealth had introduced the Casemix Development Programme as part of its Medicare agreement with the states to establish systems and parameters for the use of casemix classification systems within Australia.

PUBLIC/PRIVATE SECTOR BLURRING

Whilst the private hospital sector had a long history in Australia, interest in public sector technical efficiency led to an increasing interest in a range of private health sector roles. Health planners began to become involved in experimentation in providing health care in the private sector so as to develop competitive markets, improve efficiency (for example, through substitutability) and, in line with the current trends, develop ways of shifting costs from the public capped system to the private uncapped system. Such approaches included planning for primary care treatment centres attached to public hospitals, planning for day surgeries and contracting out services such as pathology and radiology.

In the 1980s, state governments legislated for greater planning and regulatory control of private hospitals. The Private Health Establishments Act was passed in New South Wales in 1982 and proclaimed in 1988. Similar legislation was passed in Victoria in 1982. These Acts provided for a planned development of private services. Licensing of hospitals would be subject to planning guidelines.

A DOSE OF EQUITY

In the 1980s, initially with support from the Whitlam Labour government and with the development of civil rights movements internationally, interest groups began to emerge as political and policy forces in Australia. Health interest groups concerned with mental health, ageing and disability and other particular health issues developed or moved from a charitable emphasis to become advocacy groups. Specific health services — such as Aboriginal medical services, women's health centres, community mental health and disability services, women's refuges, rape crisis centres and ethno-specific health workers and interpreters — were funded to address equity and access issues. Access and equity plans and policies designed to overcome access barriers began to be considered by Commonwealth and state bureaucracies.

INTEGRATED HEALTH SERVICES PLANNING DEVELOPS

Decentralisation was a key strategy of the 1980s to promote health services that were responsive to community needs, if not to incorporate community participation mechanisms. The effect of the regional- or area-based organisation was that planning for super-speciality services began to be undertaken at the central or national level, planning for secondary and primary care services was undertaken at the area/regional level and operational or business planning was undertaken at the local level. During this period, specialist planners were appointed at the central and regional/area tiers of administration and occasionally at the local level.

Systemic issues which began to be evaluated and addressed included: the level of integration of hospital and community care; the historical patterns of service delivery; traditional hospital management structures as compared to more 'responsive' area and regional structures; population locational access and equity issues, particularly as they related to hospital facilities; the possible range of private health sector roles; and the need for information tools to more effectively assess health service outputs. These systemic changes in health care management were accompanied later in the 1980s by interest in health care quality and in epidemiology. By the end of the 1980s the public health movement again began to have a voice and to provide a countervailing influence to the developing corporatist efficiency paradigm.

Changes in mental health, aged care and disability legislation and policy in the 1980s particularly supported deinstitutionalisation. The relatively large institutional or nursing home bed numbers were inappropriately concentrated in metropolitan areas, there was a lack of adequate community homes and hostel beds and, in general, there was a lack of appropriate assessment and community- and home-based alternatives. In mental health and disability services, the introduction of psychotropic drugs in the 1960s and 1970s had given impetus to community care. Important changes in mental health legislation and policy occurred during the 1980s, such that mental illness was legally redefined and procedures were improved for involuntary incarceration, as were mechanisms for appeal and review.

This range of legislative, human rights, treatment improvement and cost consideration changes led to a considerable shift in the numbers of people being institutionalised.

There was considerable activity in service planning, variously supported by policies and programme funding designed to develop more integrated community-based service models. Questions about the level of community resources required for community-based treatment, rehabilitation, palliation and care were frequently raised.

STATES START TO ACT ON LOCATIONAL EQUITY

During the 1980s the planning processes highlighted locational inequity in many states. In some states, historical spending patterns were questioned through the use of needs-based indicators and early resource allocation formulae.

In New South Wales, for example, the Minister for Health, the Hon. Kevin Stewart, announced in 1979 the closure of 879 hospital beds in Sydney and 1200 in rural New South Wales and the redistribution of the savings to growth areas. In 1983 the NSW Minister for Health, the Hon. Laurie Brereton, further announced the closure of two medium-sized hospitals and the downgrading of the Sydney and War Memorial Hospitals in order to fund beds in Sydney's rapidly growing western suburbs. These latter changes created much greater furore than the previous closures. Such redistributions also occurred to a lesser extent in Melbourne and Adelaide and they continue today as major themes in hospital services planning.

PLANNING TOOLS DEVELOP

Health planners gradually began to be involved in developing sophisticated technical approaches to forecasting needs and trends. In the mid-1980s, role delineation of services was developed as a planning process. Role delineation of health services allowed planners and managers to assess the support services, staffing profile, minimal safety standards and other requirements for each health care service and facility. Role delineation supported the provision of specific services outside of the hospital grounds in a more efficient or effective networked arrangement. Making such clinical requirements explicit provided a more consistent way of ensuring that patients received safe care in the most appropriate facility and service.

By the late 1980s, computer modelling became firmly established. In 1985 a forecasting model was used by the Western Metropolitan Health Region of New South Wales. This set the framework for the development of teaching facilities and further redistribution of hospital beds, within the region. In the early 1990s, HOSPIM, a locational optimisation model, was used for metropolitan hospital planning in South Australia; the Victorians developed HOSPLOC, a simulation model, for reconfiguring metropolitan hospital services; and New South Wales developed the APPI Planner. In Western Australia the epidemiological contribution to planning was enhanced in the mid-1990s through record linkage of six main health databases.

DEVELOPMENT OF SPECIALISED PLANNING

The increasing use of technologies and the use of high-cost drugs in the 1970s contributed to higher health costs. Unlike other industries, where technology reduces costs, most medical technology has not been labour displacing and often results in the creation of additional jobs. Health technology planning was begun in earnest by a sub-committee of the Standing Committee of Health Ministers (SCOHM), a predecessor to the Australian Health Ministers Advisory Committee (AHMAC). Planning ratios for services such as cardiac surgery, renal dialysis and computer tomography (CT) scanners were all issues of concern.

The application of these ratios at the state level was not easy, due to political lobbying for new and expansive technology. In the 1980s, Victoria put into legislation a planning approach to regulate the diffusion of CT scanners, linear accelerators, lithotripters and Magnetic Resonance Imaging (MRIs), whereby a need had to be demonstrated before licence would be granted. Enshrining technology planning into legislation was ultimately abandoned in the 1990s when placing financial limitations — either through Commonwealth payments or through national pooled funding via AHMAC — on technology diffusion became the preferred approach. Magnetic resonance imaging and transplantations (heart, liver, lung and pancreas) were the primary targets of funding restrictions during the early 1990s.

Health manpower (sic) planning began in earnest at both state and Commonwealth levels when AHMAC was asked to report on an 'oversupply' of doctors. The supply of doctors had increased in the 1970s due to the expansion of medical schools, as recommended by the Karmel report into medical education. Furthermore, from the 1960s, 'foreign doctors' or overseas- trained doctors gradually began to be licensed to practise in various states.

Since then, workforce planning has re-emerged at times when workforce issues have been characterised by tensions between specialisation and multiskilling, or due to contests between different professional groups (especially medicine and nursing), perceived tensions between equity principles such as equal employment opportunity (EEO) and the efficiency drive and an emerging concern with professional standards and quality care.

During the 1980s the medical profession regularly went to battle with various governments and the bureaucracy on issues which included pharmaceutical benefits, staffing of community health centres, health insurance, registration of alternative health care practitioners, medical fees and the differential between general practitioner and specialist charges. Medicare had resulted in declining revenues for hospitals and for some private physicians. These factors contributed to the development of a 'festering and periodically explosive doctor' dispute' from 1984 onwards.

In the 1990s the battles between the medical profession and governments resulted in medical workforce planning as a process to negotiate the supply of specialist doctors. The Australian Medical Workforce Advisory Council (AMWAC), a sub-committee of AHMAC, is the forum where representatives of the various specialities come to agreement about shortages and oversupplies and how these might be addressed.

The recruitment and retention of nurses, allied health and a number of other health disciplines also emerged as problems from time to time throughout the 1970s and 1980s. The fluctuations in these workforce categories reflected more the position of women in the economy and workforce.

The 1980s also heralded significant changes in the nursing profession. Since the Second World War, nursing had been beset with recurring labour shortages, poor remuneration, inadequate training and poor working conditions. The patient care context for nursing had significantly shifted, such that individual nurses rather than just the hospital matron (as under the Nightingale system) now had responsibility to independently solve clinical problems. This led inevitably to tensions between greater specialisation and multiskilling in nursing. During the 1980s, nurses' wages and conditions improved and the gradual transfer of nurse education from the hospital setting to the higher education sector provided for increasing professionalism. These changes also increased the overall costs of health care, since nursing labour represented about half the total costs of health care.

With involvement in workforce planning issues, planning moved beyond its role of the early 1980s when designated health planners had mainly been involved in developing service and strategic plans for the health system. By the end of the 1980s, in keeping with the rise of managerialism at that time, corporate and business plans derived from the US private sector began to be fashionable.

These plans differed from previous strategic plans in that they defined goals, objectives and strategies for the whole organisation. Planning's corporate role became intimately tied up with its service planning role. The first state corporate plan was developed in Western Australia in 1986. In 1989 the Western Australia Strategic Plan for the Health Department fully integrated the previous corporate, strategic and service plans. Corporate plans were developed in the late 1980s and early 1990s in most other states.

RATIONING, EFFECTIVENESS AND OUTCOMES

In the 1990s, planning moved from a concern with inputs to a concern with outcomes. This movement signalled a change of focus, from measuring the services that are provided to measuring the health gain achieved from those services. An outcome focus in planning related to issues surrounding quality management, the establishment of national health goals and targets and an interest in outcome evaluation.

This shift was also consistent with the move of the planning role into organisational management and improving performance monitoring and accountability. Planning became increasingly concerned with resource allocation issues, or with organisational, capital or service planning which required an 'outcomes focus' or a focus on 'health improvement'.

Whilst a traditional service planning approach allowed planners to retreat to data collection, sophisticated forecasting and computer modelling, the health outcomes approach required evidence of relative need, knowledge of the best available evidence of the effectiveness of interventions and evidence of appropriate community, intersectoral and stakeholder consultation. It incorporated an economic component and required integrated planning processes.

At one level the outcomes paradigm provided a new set of principles on which to ration health care — merely another way for administrators to take control of the knife, wield it and then justify its use. At another level, in combination with improved information systems, the outcomes approach had potential to further challenge traditional practices and routines in health care and to develop more cost-effective, patient/community-centred and broad- based approaches to improving health.

The adoption of 'evidence-based medicine' began to be advocated both for clinical practice and in policy and planning. Such an approach required the planning process to take account of the findings of research and data and to develop skills in analysing effectiveness, safety and acceptability, the quality of evidence and the generalisability and local applicability of research and data. The outcomes movement contributed to increasing involvement of frontline health workers in clinical research, business planning and information gathering.

At the same time, designated planning units were often abandoned in favour of private consultants or market forces. Where planning was totally abandoned in favour of market forces, a commitment to distributional equity was also substantially abandoned.

Policy and planning documents became replete with both the language of economic rationalism and the public health and health outcomes lexicon. Tensions between public health and biomedicine, between outputs and outcomes and between planning and market forces characterised the health planning environment.

Whereas in the previous decade the planning process could often be topdown, the public health approach and market assessment required a more rigourous and intersectoral approach to needs assessment and applied epidemiology.

Health planning required a more eclectic approach that integrated processes which had previously been discrete and sequential, including service planning, economic appraisal and capital and asset planning. Planning was essentially concerned with change management and economics. Planning also became a skill expected of most health care managers and administrators.

THE FUTURE OF HEALTH PLANNING

The future is likely to see further cost restraint, new approaches to resource allocation, the predicted ageing of the population, the predicted ethical and financial difficulties for the health care system of delivering equitable services to the 'old old', an increase in technology and new treatments, a further blurring of the public and private components of health care and greater community and consumer involvement in health care.

Key questions for the system are whether to focus resources on improving the health of 'the many' (equity of access), or to focus resources, activities and interventions on those with the poorest health, thereby attempting to equalise their health outcomes with those of the rest of the population (equity of outcome). Questions must also arise as to whether health services and facilities remain at the forefront of health planning activity, or whether broader social and intersectoral approaches become pivotal.

Certainly, the current political, economic and scientific environment is replete with individualistic approaches to prevention and treatment issues. The march of bio-medical approaches to health care and health improvement remains strong and constant. A reductionist approach to improving health is ever more likely as scientists and the general community become increasingly fascinated with genetics, genetic manipulation and molecular approaches to improving health. Public health has been identified as being at the crossroads, with the inevitable clash of reductionist and broad visions of health. As health planning develops the change mechanisms that are consistent with prevailing outcomes policy paradigms, it is also at a crossroads, with individualistic, top-down approaches down one road and intersectoral, inclusive, health improvement and equity planning down the other.

❐

Chapter - 4

Impact of the Economy on Health Care

In the United States, the economy shapes the complex interactions among employment, health coverage and costs, and financial access to care and health outcomes. The effects of economic stress and surges can be observed directly, but may also surface in less obvious ways that can vary markedly across markets. In a system where employment-based coverage plays a dominant role, understanding the impact of economic shocks such as the current recession presents difficult analytical issues.

An off-the-record, facilitated discussion conducted under the Robert Wood Johnson Foundation's Changes in Health Care Financing and Organization (HCFO) Initiative provided impetus for planning new research to explore the interconnections among economic forces, health care access, costs, and outcomes. The session began a discussion about what we know, how comprehensive reforms may transform the health care landscape in the United States, and what can be done to increase our capacity to address vitally important policy questions about health care and population health in the wake of the worst recession ever experienced by the great majority of our population.

THE ECONOMY, EMPLOYMENT, AND HEALTH COVERAGE

Over the past two decades, there have been, in addition to a variety of downswings and recoveries, three "official" recessions, based on the criteria applied by the National Bureau of Economic Research (NBER): one in the early 1990s (lasting eight months); one in 2001 (lasting eight months) and the current recession, which officially began in December 2007, and is by far the most extensive contraction since the Great Depression.

Throughout the past 20 years, employer-sponsored health insurance has been the dominant source of coverage for the non-elderly population, backed up, in various ways, by public policies designed to protect people who lose their jobs, primarily the Consolidated Omnibus Budget Reconciliation Act (COBRA), with some additional support from other federal legislation, including the Health Insurance Portability and Accountability Act (HIPAA), and by public programmes that provide health coverage to low income populations, mainly Medicaid and the Children's Health Insurance Programme (CHIP).

During this same period, there have been significant changes in the design of health benefits and cost-sharing available in the group and individual insurance markets, as well as in public programmes.

RECESSIONS AND EMPLOYMENT-BASED COVERAGE

Unemployment data from the Bureau of Labour Statistics' Current Population Survey showed that the unemployment rate in the United States was 9.5 per cent in June 2009, more than double the rate of 4.6 per cent in June 2007. The loss of jobs in the current recession, as in previous recessions and other, less profound economic downturns is clearly associated with reductions in health coverage.

Analysis conducted for the Kaiser Family Foundation in 2002 showed that in the previous decade, including the recession in 2001, every percentage point increase in the unemployment rate leads to an increase of 0.5 percentage point in the non-elderly population without health insurance. The Urban Institute, in an analysis of more recent data, estimates that a 1.0 percentage point increase in the unemployment rate results in a 0.59 percentage point increase in the share of non-elderly adults without insurance.

Recession leads almost immediately to loss of coverage for many individuals and their families who were insured through employer arrangements. While newly unemployed workers may be able to retain coverage temporarily, others will not qualify for or cannot afford continuation coverage under COBRA or other available programmes. COBRA continuation coverage does not extend to employees enrolled in group insurance plans provided by employers with fewer than 20 employees, nor to those covered by employers who declare bankruptcy and discontinue all health plans.

Additional reductions in coverage are triggered by employers' needs to control benefit costs when the economy contracts. Economists argue that employee benefit costs are traded off against wages, so that decreasing benefits is not an effective way of limiting costs. But there are also real economic costs associated with the administration of benefits programmes, and still other costs associated with cutting benefits, such as lower employee morale.

While perceptions about the economics of employer-sponsored health benefits may differ, the outcome appears to be that most employers who have been able to offer health coverage are reluctant to eliminate health insurance benefits entirely, even during severe economic downturns. Research examining the relationships among economic cycles and costs of employee coverage in the late 1980s and early 1990s found that rather than dropping insurance benefits altogether, employers generally responded to the pressures of economic downturns by shifting premium costs to employees. Rates of employer-sponsored coverage did not, however, return to pre-recession levels in the recovery that followed the recession in the first part of this decade.

Analysis of declines in health coverage in the 1990s also found that the overall level of health coverage fell even when the economy was thriving, as a growing percentage of employees who could elect to receive benefits opted not to when their premium costs continued to increase. The 2008 Health Research and Education Trust (HRET) survey of employers found—even at the onset of what turned out to be a major recession—that among those firms offering health benefits, few reported that they were "very likely" to drop coverage or restrict employee eligibility in the coming year. More commonly, employers intended to find ways to reduce their costs by changing benefits and cost-sharing provisions. A survey of 438 employers conducted in March 2009 found, for example, that close to half were planning to make more cost- saving changes to health benefits than usual in response to economic conditions, including the adoption of consumer-driven plans (generally high- deductible plans with health savings accounts) or other high-deductible options, as well as tightening up on administrative costs, vendor payments, and dependent eligibility determinations.

Measuring the full extent of the current recession on insurance coverage is not possible in "real time." Reductions in health insurance coverage lag behind job loss due to the temporary continuation of coverage available to some employees, and because changes in employer coverage are generally implemented in annual contracts.

In addition, some people who lose employment-based coverage are able, after some lapse in coverage, to obtain new coverage from other sources, including public programmes for low-income families or veterans, or to obtain coverage through a spouse, or through the individual market. The American Recovery and Reinvestment Act (ARRA) of 2009 (the "stimulus package") provides a subsidy to unemployed workers eligible for COBRA, such that eligible individuals are required to pay only 35 per cent of the premiums for COBRA, (rather than the usual 100 per cent) as well as certain state and local coverage continuation programmes, for up to nine months.

The effects of the subsidy on laid-off employees' election of COBRA benefits are not yet known. The 2009 Spencer's Benefit Report survey of employers found that, prior to the subsidies, fewer than one in five laid-off employees had elected COBRA coverage, primarily because the premium costs were too high. The capacity of public programmes—Medicaid and CHIP, Veterans Health Administration, the Indian Health Service, federally funded community health centers, and state and local programmes—to fill in the gaps in coverage is limited. A study completed in early 2009 found that only 1 in 4 unemployed workers age 16 to 65 who had incomes below 200 per cent of poverty received health coverage through Medicaid or other public programmes. With the additional federal funding provided in the 2009 CHIP reauthorization, some states expanded coverage for children or pregnant women. But other financially strapped states have been unable to come up with their share of the funds needed to expand CHIP coverage, and some, including California, have had to freeze CHIP eligibility. Pressure on public programmes may not only restrict coverage and reduce benefits available to low-income unemployed families, but also add displaced public health workers and employees who administer the public programmes to the unemployment rolls.

Determining the appropriate frames for comparison can be subjective. Is the relevant issue "What will happen to health coverage going forward, as the economy recovers?" or "How has insurance coverage changed in response to this recession compared to what might have been had the recession been less severe?" Significant numbers of laid-off workers were not covered by employer-sponsored plans.

Employees in low-wage jobs, those working in small firms, and those in certain industries have been far more likely than others to have been uninsured when they lost their jobs. But this time, those losing their jobs as the recession deepened have been working in industries or firms (for example, finance) that have generally provided generous health benefits. Retiree coverage could also be in play in some sectors of the economy. Shedding costs for retirees' health coverage or for Medicare supplemental coverage and/or prescription drug coverage could be important for firms facing bankruptcy.

Determining how economic recession affects insurance coverage therefore needs to take a variety of factors into account, including what types of jobs, with what levels and generosity of insurance benefits, are lost, and what other forms of coverage are available to different populations. The Urban Institute study includes separate estimates for children and non-elderly adults, broken down to show the interrelated effects on coverage generated by changes in enrollment in employer-sponsored coverage, Medicaid/CHIP, and non-group coverage. The study estimates that moving from the baseline rate of 4.6 per cent unemployment in 2007 to a rate of 10 per cent unemployment would result in 13.2 million fewer people with employer-sponsored health coverage, offset by an increase of 5.4 million enrolling in Medicaid and CHIP and 1.8 million in non-group coverage; altogether, about 5.8 million more non-elderly adults and children would become uninsured.

STRUCTURAL TRENDS

While employment-based health insurance is obviously strained by economic contractions, there are also broader factors shaping the scope of coverage of American workers and their families. Structural changes in insurance coverage and in the economy over time are particularly salient. First, while employer-sponsored coverage has maintained its dominant role in health coverage, the design and cost of employer-sponsored coverage has changed, leading to a decline in the rate at which employees are choosing, or are able, to take up insurance offers.

Second, more people are finding work in jobs that are less likely to offer comprehensive health benefits. Because coverage depends on where people find jobs as well as on whether those jobs include health insurance benefits, employer-sponsored coverage may be less secure over time.

Employer-sponsored coverage has, from one perspective, proven to be quite resilient. The percentage of employers offering health benefits has been relatively stable over the past decade; most large and medium-sized firms offer health benefits, and, even among small firms (fewer than 200 workers) the percentage offering heath coverage has been relatively stable. HRET survey data show that in 1999, 99 per cent of large firms and 65 per cent of all small firms offered health benefits; in 2008, 99 per cent of large firms and 62 per cent of small firms offered benefits.

Note, however, that there was a large fall in employer-sponsored insurance sponsorship rates, larger for small firms, between 2001 and 2005, and that over this period, low-income workers were more likely to lose employer- sponsored coverage than higher-income workers. The longer period, including both good and bad years, may average out coverage rates over the cycle.

Nevertheless, in the face of rising health care costs, employers have continued to look for ways to redesign insurance coverage. Economic contractions may have increased the urgency of employers' cost containment efforts, and may have made it easier to overcome employee resistance to changes. But because health care costs have increased faster than wages or general inflation in good economic times as well as bad, changes in benefit design are not likely to be reversed when the economy turns around.

For example, the recession in the early 1990s may have provided additional impetus to employer efforts to control costs by moving away from indemnity models to managed care plans. The recession in 2001 came on the heels of employers' retreat from managed care approaches that engendered public back-lash; employers opted instead to increase employee cost-sharing requirements. In the current recession, employers appear to be increasing their attention on consumer-driven options, but also on health promotion activities and other changes to benefits that might help to reduce utilization of health services.

These emerging interests may also be reinforced by possible national health reform initiatives on health promotion and disease prevention. From the perspective of most employees, however, the most salient trend over the past decade has been an increase in the costs of premiums and growing levels of cost sharing, including higher copayments and coinsurance. In particular, more low-wage workers are opting not to take up coverage that is increasingly expensive.

Because the costs borne by employees as well as the availability of coverage varies widely across regions, industries, and establishment size, longer-term changes in the economy are intertwined with changes in insurance design. More workers employed in low-wage, temporary, part-time work, and a shift to jobs in retail and service sectors industries may contribute to less affordable, less comprehensive employer-sponsored coverage for a growing segment of the working population.

These shifts can be either cyclical or structural. Analysis of the Community Tracking Study (CTS), for example, found that economic cycles affect the "quality" of jobs, including whether they offer health insurance. Over the longer term, however, permanent shifts in the industrial base could change the dynamics of employment-based coverage. For example, the effects of a restructured auto industry, historically among the most important players in the employer-sponsored insurance market, could yield important insights.

Small firms also play a critical role in the longer-term structure of employment-based coverage. About half of all paid employees (across all industries) worked in enterprises with fewer than 500 employees (2006 data); about 18 per cent worked in private sector enterprises with fewer than 20 employees.

In expanding as well as contracting econo mies, small employers are less able to find affordable coverage for employees and, in many cases, have limited resources to organize or manage health benefits or to subsidize benefit costs. Small businesses also represent a "permanently changing" segment of the workforce. About 8 of 10 new establishments survive for a full year, and 2 in 3 survive two years, and less than half survive four years.

The entry and exit of hundreds of thousands of new businesses each year, most of which begin with a very small number of employees, also limit the ability of these establishments to provide stable coverage (and also greatly complicates the task of analysing coverage trends).

THE ECONOMY, HEALTH PROVIDERS, AND MARKETS

The health care industry is a critical component of the national, and most regional and local economies in the United States. Cyclical economic contractions, innovations in medical technology, shifts in public policy, and local market factors can result in different, and sometimes contradictory, pressures on the supply and organization of health care delivery systems, suppliers, and practitioners.

RECESSION AND HEALTH CARE DELIVERY

The effects of economic shifts include changes in the demand for (or access to) health care, but also organizations' and practitioners' own financial status. Reports from markets across the United States are describing a sort of perfect storm: falling revenues due to decreased demand for less non-urgent or elective care, more patients unable to pay their medical bills, significant losses in investment income, less charitable giving, and cuts in health care funding by states and localities.

A survey conducted by the American Academy of Family Physicians received only a very small number of responses from the 10,000 physicians polled, but among those who did respond, more than half reported seeing fewer patients since the recession began. A survey of community hospital CEOs fielded by the American Hospital Association (AHA) in March 2009 also reported that fewer patients were seeking inpatient and elective services.

At the same time, physicians and institutional providers report seeing more patients without insurance, or with inadequate insurance, who are unable to pay for their care. Some providers have compensated for lost revenue by expanding their hours of operation. Many, however, report that they are dealing with declining volume and lost revenues from unpaid bills by reducing services or cutting staff. The AHA 2009 survey of community hospitals found that 9 in 10 had made some cuts in response to economic concerns, including reducing staff or administrative expenses, or reducing services. Many reported scaling back on capital improvements, including putting upgrades to clinical and information technology systems on hold. Survey respondents also reported that physicians are increasingly seeking financial support such as opportunities for on-call pay or employment.

The effects of economic contractions can be hard to parse out because they run counter to the sustained growth in the health sector. Rather than an actual contraction, the recession may have resulted in a slower growth of health care-related jobs overall. Some of the fastest-growing employment in health care has been jobs such as therapists, aides, technicians, and personal care assistants, which are distributed throughout both the private and public sectors of the economy. Cost-cutting by hospitals or by public programmes struggling with budget deficits could slow the growth of these jobs, but perhaps only temporarily.

At the same time, the recession has increased demand for care in community settings that provide subsidized or low-cost care. Many community health centers, for example, have reported a surge in the number of new uninsured people seeking care. Funding from the federal stimulus bill directed to community health centers should help meet some of their growing needs, but at the same time cutbacks in state funding reduce resources for community health centers as well as safety net hospitals. Determining the net effect of the recession on health care jobs may therefore be difficult.

The recession has also created pressure on health care professionals to revise their career and retirement plans. There is some evidence that employment of registered nurses grows during economic downturns. A recent analysis suggested that concerns about family income, for example a spouse being laid off, lead nurses to reenter the job market. There are also reports that nurses may be delaying retirement. At the same time, retrenchment by health providers reduced the number of nursing job openings in some market segments.

In the Boston area, for example, staff reductions associated with a downturn in elective hospital admissions, combined with a growing number of nurses seeking to go back to work, resulted in a shortage of job openings for nurses for the first time in years. Some analysts fear that the temporary rush into the labour market will be followed by mass exits when the economy recovers, intensifying a longer-standing nursing shortage

This recession may also impact physicians more significantly than previous, less severe economic downturns. Physicians who have lost significant amounts of their investment portfolios may be postponing their retirement, either by continuing in their current practice longer than they had planned, or by establishing practice arrangements with hospitals or other provider groups. Physician leaders have also expressed concern that students seeking loans for medical school education might not be able to find them in the distressed credit market.

In the short term, physicians' need to remain in the workforce could possibly offset a predicted shortage or primary care doctors. But if older physicians are concerned about generating revenue to replace investment losses, and younger cohorts are saddled with excessive debt, economic incentives to practice in more lucrative subspecialties could become even more persuasive, further exacerbating the pressure on primary care

STRUCTURAL TRENDS

Over the longer term, factors such as a growing demand for health care, more formal or virtual integration of services delivery facilitated by health information technology, or substantive legislative reforms affecting the financing and regulation of heath care could overwhelm the effects of economic cycles.

Two dominant trends—growth and consolidation—are likely to continue to reshape health care delivery, but reform legislation, related changes in federal investment in health information technology and health manpower, and provider payment could significantly affect the direction of changes. Horizontal and vertical integration of providers might be accelerated by recession, but the trend can also be seen as a response to longer term pressures.

A surge in hospital mergers and acquisitions in the 1990s was driven by structural changes including technologies that moved services to outpatient settings. Consolidations provided hospital systems with an opportunity to enhance and better leverage their market positions. Over time the prevalence of independent practitioners has also been declining. Data from the CTS shows that the percentage of primary care physicians in independent practices declined by 5 percentage points from 1996-97 to 2004-05, while the percentage of medical specialists and surgical specialists in independent practices declined 19 percentage points and 9 percentage points, respectively. Much of the change is the result of physicians moving to mid- sized single specialty groups. Physician groups were also focused on increasing efficiency and containing costs before the onset of the credit crisis that ushered in the current recession.

Looking forward, major insurance and financing reforms could change the incentives driving provider restructuring in different sectors of the health industry.

Significant increases in coverage of previously uninsured or underinsured populations could reshape the demand for services. Changes in insurance regulation, along with payment reforms, could shift the incentives that drive providers' decisions about where and when they want to work. Comprehensive coverage reforms could lead to restructuring the roles of safety net providers and a redistribution of uncompensated care funding to a broader set of providers. Other reforms designed to promote the effectiveness and quality of health care, including increased funding and technical assistance for the implementation of health information and clinical management systems, could accelerate movement of independent practitioners into integrated systems. How structural changes will play out across different markets and what these might mean for the delivery of care for different populations will present very difficult challenges to the research community.

THE ECONOMY AND POPULATION HEALTH

Although economic factors clearly affect the use of health services and health outcomes, the interactions among access, health-related behaviour, and use of health services can be difficult to sort out. Variation in demographic and other factors across regions and markets make measuring the effects of economic forces even more difficult.

RECESSIONS, HEALTH UTILIZATION, AND OUTCOMES

Unemployment, lower income, or losing insurance coverage in economic downturns can result in reduced access to health services. Economic uncertainty itself also affects people's behaviour, including how they spend money on health care and on other commodities or activities that can affect their health and health outcomes. Various reports suggest that the current recession is leading some to forego not just elective surgery and preventive screenings, but also basic care for acute and chronic conditions.

One privately-funded panel survey of more that 100,000 households found a marked increase in the percentage of households reporting that they had deferred (delayed or cancelled) health visits in early 2009, compared to 2006. The most commonly deferred care was physician visits (54.7 per cent); followed by imaging procedures (8 per cent), non-elective procedures (6.2 per cent), and lab or diagnostic tests (5.7 per cent). Deferring care was most prominent in lower-income households, but occurred across all income and age cohorts.

A survey of employees who were [still] employed and insured through employer-sponsored or union-sponsored plans found evidence that the recession was taking a toll on employees' physical and emotional health: 27 per cent reported that they had chosen not to receive health care treatment to save money on coinsurance or copayments, 20 per cent had skipped taking medications at the prescribed dosage, 17 per cent were splitting drug dosages to make them last longer, and 40 per cent said their mental health/stress/ anxiety levels had become worse since the economic downturn. Available evidence regarding the immediate versus longer-term effects of economic downturns and recovery on population health is somewhat ambiguous, however.

For example, there is some evidence that economic pressure may lead more women to seek reproductive services, and, in particular, long-term contraception, and abortions.

At the same time, there is some evidence suggesting that, at least in previous recessions, decreased access to or use of prenatal services has been associated with a higher incident of adverse pregnancy outcomes such as anemia and low-birth weight infants in some low-income populations. More recently, researchers have focused attention on an apparent link between recessions, reduced industrial pollution, lower levels of particulates in the atmosphere, and lower rates of infant mortality. A body of economic research focused more broadly on the effects of economic cycles on health perhaps raises as many questions as it answers.

A number of studies have found that health outcomes, as measured by mortality rates, are counter-cyclical, that is, mortality rates are worse (higher) when the economy gets better. Explanations for this phenomenon generally focus on factors that could increase mortality in active economies, such as more deaths from traffic accidents because more people are commuting to work or taking vacations; more industrial production, increasing pollution as well as the probability of accidents; more cardiovascular illness related to work- related stress; or, changes in behaviour during recessions that could reduce mortality rates, such as being more careful about eating, exercise, alcohol use, etc. when money is tight.

Research examining some of these possible explanations again presents a complex picture. A review of studies examining the effects of physician strikes shows that mortality rates go down when elective surgeries are less available. But while some research has linked recessions to lower mortality rates for cardiovascular disease, economic downturns have also been linked to markedly higher rates of cancer deaths and homicides, and to a wide range of psychiatric disorders, as well as alcohol and substance abuse. Although researchers have suggested that people may be more careful about diet and lifestyle when they are worried about money, there is also some evidence that the opposite may occur as well.

A survey conducted by the American Heart Association in March 2009 found that about a third of respondents had made changes over the preceding 6 months that could have negative health consequences, including delaying preventive care appointments, not taking medications, or skipping dental appointments; 42 per cent said they planned to make changes in the coming months that could be detrimental to their health, such as buying fewer fruits and vegetables. Research examining the effects of a recession in the early 1900s found that higher rates of cardiovascular disease contributed to a 15 month shorter lifespan for those born during the recession compared to people born into a healthier economy. Although the applicability of these findings in the very different environment of the 21st century is questionable, more current work relating birth weight to economic conditions suggests that many unanswered questions remain about the effect of suboptimal conditions on early childhood development and longer-term health outcomes.

STRUCTURAL CHANGES

The demand for health care and the benefits it brings have continued, rarely abated, over the past half century. The demand for health care is expected to continue to increase, accounting for a significantly larger proportion of the national economy. But as the importance of health care and its costs has grown, systemic problems affecting different subgroups of the population have become intertwined with the economic forces affecting access, costs, and outcomes. Data from the National Health Interview Survey from 1997 through 2008 show a generally increasing trend in the percentage of people who reported that they failed to receive needed medical care due to cost over the course of the year. Failing to get care was more prevalent among those aged 18-64, and higher among Hispanic and non-Hispanic black persons. The percentage of people reporting that they had a regular place to go for medical care generally decreased, as did the percentage of people who said they had excellent or very good health.

A variety of factors are increasing the need for health care. For example, the prevalence of obesity among U.S. adults aged 20 and older has generally increased over time, from 19.4 per cent in 1997 to 27.6 per cent in the last quarter of 2008.

Major reforms to the current system that would ensure that most Americans would have comprehensive health insurance, and be able to retain it even when there are major economic contractions, would almost certainly moderate the variability of health care access and utilization over economic cycles. Delivery system reforms, such as investments in primary care, health information systems, or evidence-based clinical management systems could also help address systemic problems associated with accessing needed health care.

LOOKING AHEAD

To understand the effects of economic shifts, it is critical to sort out cyclical effects of the economy on health coverage, utilization, and the structure and efficiency of health care delivery from longer term structural changes. Some changes to the employment base—such as bankruptcies or reductions in force that also eliminate employees' access to health coverage, or cuts in employer investments in insurance—may turn around as the economy cycles back up.

Other effects of downturns, or adjustments in the structure of employment during recoveries, may involve changes not likely to be reversed, or may affect the trajectory of longer term trends, or perhaps move health care in entirely new directions.

Changes in insurance coverage or in provider organization may also affect different segments of the population differently, contributing to longer term effects on health outcomes.

The analytical challenges arising from this complexity are exacerbated by the lack of data needed to understand how insurance coverage, financial access to care, and the use of health services changes over the course of economic cycles among different populations.

While there is a vast body of research to support future analysis of economic forces on health care and health, the breadth of changes that could be set in motion by comprehensive reform legislation will add complexity. It will be important to understand, for example, how reforms might affect providers' ability to meet the demands of a better-insured population, including decisions about health professionals' and provider organizations' market participation; how changes in insurance regulation and enrollment in private and public insurance plans affects the distribution of insurance risk; how different insurance plans or care delivery systems are able to work with health practitioners and with consumers to improve the efficiency and quality of care delivery; and how well changes driven by the reforms actually work to improve health care access, efficiencies, and outcomes.

The current literature also demonstrates the limitations of efforts, drawn from assorted analyses of a very complex puzzle, to understand of how economic forces effect health care access, utilization, quality, and costs. To evaluate reforms, or to understand the full impact of failing to make changes to the health care coverage and delivery systems, researchers will need to draw on more complete data than is now readily available. This would include data that link people, their employers, their insurance coverage, their health care utilization, costs, and health outcomes, and how these interrelated factors change over time and across different populations.
❐

Chapter - 5

Marketing in Health Care

HEALTH MARKETING

Health marketing is a new approach to public health that applies traditional marketing principles and theories alongside science-based strategies toprevention, health promotion and health protection. Health marketing is one of the ways through which advancements in medicine and in health- protecting services like insurance are made widely known. A good example is the current drive in Kenya to promote circumcision among communities that do not customarily circumcise. Medical researchers have recently documented that circumcision is 65% effective in preventing HIV infection among men.

The marketing strategy would follow the traditional 4 "P's" of marketing namely:

- The "product" in question in this case the surgical procedure.
- The "place" which refers to the access to this procedure.
- "Promotion" refers to creating awareness and hence demand.
- "Price" refers to the cost of the procedure e.g. money, time, reputation etc.

"Health marketing" is a term rarely used in public health and related disciplines. "Social marketing" or "integrated marketing communication" are more commonly used in public health and other disciplines to refer to marketing-based planning frameworks for public health communication.

HEALTH CARE MARKETING PLAN

Assessment: Consult business plans, patient satisfaction surveys, volume reports, community surveys and any other information you can gather. Consider market dynamics such as seasonality, shifting alliances between physician groups and other "political" issues. Comparative analysis: Study your competitors, considering their historical advertising levels, any new product launches that may be forthcoming, and the overall competitive nature of your market. Develop your own "unique selling proposition." What makes you different from your competition?

Define your vision and strategy: Where do you want your programme or organization to be in three to five years? How can marketing help realize this vision? Make a list of all the tools at your disposal and determine what options will work best for your product, marketplace and expected budget.

Among other tools, consider:

- Networking/sales—Go where your market is; develop presentations.
- Direct marketing—Use letters, fliers, brochures, postcards.
- Advertising—Consider print, broadcast, outdoor, special publications such as chamber of commerce directories and sports programmes.
- Training programmes—Increase awareness of your services by offering training to your customers.
- Free media—Write articles for news media; make your organization known as the expert.
- Public relations—Consider sponsorships that "fit" with your service; hold events, tours, open houses.
- Web site/emerging media—It's not just for young professionals anymore; fast-growing segments of the elderly and minority populations are using the Internet to gather information on their health care options.

Build support and enthusiasm: Locate your champions in the organization. Find the experts who will help support your marketing efforts through speaking engagements, newspaper interviews, and quotes for newsletters and media releases.

Segment your market: Consider target audiences and think outside the box. Look inward first, as your employees can be some of your best customers— and your best marketers. Know where your business comes from: Is it driven by physician referrals or do patients refer directly? Make a list of target audiences and identify the best ways to reach them.

Budget: Now that you have the tools you need and have determined the best way to reach your target audiences, build your budget to support the campaign. Stick with the 80/20 rule: 80 percent of your volumes will often come from 20 percent of your customers. Focus on the top group or groups to make sure your plans have the greatest impact. Determine what you can do in-house and what you need to outsource.

Build your creative: Turn your ideas into the creative product that will support your plan. Keep referring to your vision and strategy to ensure that the creative concepts support your ultimate objectives. When outsourcing, give your agency as much information as you can gather. Always share your vision.

Kick it off right: Introduce your campaign internally first. Tell physicians, employees, volunteers, board members and other stakeholders. They are often your best marketing support. Conversely, if they don't "live the message," your marketing efforts will be for naught.

Ready, set, go: Timing is everything. Plan your rollout to maximize exposure. Avoid marketplace "clutter" and down times, such as holidays, when readership and viewers are less than normal. Once you have your media plan in place, stick to it.

Measure and evaluate: Whenever possible, include a call to action that can be quantified. You may want to track new patients, calls for information, physician referrals, web site hits, patient/procedure volumes or other data meaningful to your organization. You should also consider consumer preference and top-of-mind awareness, which may translate into volumes in the future.

Whatever you do, make sure that your marketing plan becomes a part of the organizational culture. Facility plans, strategic plans and financial plans all garner the time and attention of leadership. Make sure the marketing plan is received and understood by your organization's top management.

THE EMERGING MARKET IN HEALTH CARE INNOVATION

Innovators—some from developing nations—have found ways to deliver care effectively at significantly lower cost while increasing access and quality.

Emerging innovations in the delivery of health care, particularly in developing countries, offer insights on how to tackle its rising cost, estimated at $7 trillion a year globally. Health care is consuming an escalating share of income in developed and developing nations alike. Yet innovators have found ways to deliver care effectively at significantly lower cost while improving access and increasing quality.

They are uncovering patterns for raising productivity, and leaders across health sectors—public, private, and social—should take heed. With the recent passage of health reform legislation in the United States, for instance, tackling costs is imperative there, but it is also an important goal in every other part of the world.

New approaches to the delivery of care abound. In Mexico, for example, a telephone-based health care advice and triage service is available to more than one million subscribers and their families for $5 a month, paid through phone bills. In India, an entrepreneur has proved that high-quality, no-frills maternity care can be provided for one-fifth of the price charged by the country's other private providers. In New York City, the remote monitoring of chronically ill elderly patients has reduced their rate of hospital admissions by about 40 percent.

Unfortunately, health care can be an isolated and local activity: innovations are not widely known across different systems or beyond sector boundaries. Merely identifying and promoting innovations isn't enough, however—leaders need to understand whether, and how, the lessons of innovators can be replicated elsewhere. To this end, McKinsey conducted research in partnership with the World Economic Forum to study the most promising novel forms of health care delivery and, in particular, to understand how these innovations changed its economics.

Many of the most compelling innovations we studied come not from resource-rich developed countries but from emerging markets. Two factors help explain why. First, necessity breeds innovation; in the absence of adequate health care, existing providers and entrepreneurs must improvise and innovate. Second, because of weaknesses in the infrastructure, institutions, and resources of emerging markets, entrepreneurs face fewer constraints (this is one upside of the lack of meaningful oversight, which obviously also has many drawbacks). They can bypass Western models and forge new solutions.

The nearly 30 successful innovations we looked at pursued a handful of strategies to change the economics of health care delivery in a fundamental way. In other words, they were not successful by chance. By understanding the opportunities these innovators seized, leaders throughout the health care system can identify opportunities for their own organizations.

A broad scan of innovations across the field, as well as an in-depth analysis of the business models behind 30 of them, showed us that successful ones use at least several if not all of the strategies described below.

GET CLOSE TO THE PATIENT

Innovators can lower distribution costs and improve adherence to clinical protocols by moving the delivery of care much closer to the homes of patients, providing services that take advantage of their established behaviour patterns, or both. VisionSpring, an organization that brings affordable eye care to the poor in 13 countries, succeeds because it takes care givers close to patients through a low-cost franchise model.

It teaches local "vision entrepreneurs"—members of the mainly poor communities they serve—how to diagnose problems such as presbyopia (an inability to focus on nearby objects) and how to determine what type of mass- produced eyeglass would correct it. The company also provides its entrepreneurs with a "business in a bag" that contains all the required products and equipment. Distribution costs are low because information, products, and services are standardized, and the model is simple to implement, even if the workforce is relatively unsophisticated.

USE EXISTING TECHNOLOGY TO REINVENT DELIVERY

"Repurposing" mobile-phone systems, call centers, and other existing technologies and infrastructure allows innovators to extend health care access, increase the standardization of care, and improve labour productivity. For a fixed fee of $5 a month (payable on phone bills), Mexico's MedicallHome, for example, offers its one million subscribers access to professional health advice at a cost far below the charge for a physician's visit. In Mali, Pesinet uses SMS (short message service) technology to make diagnoses of malnutrition more accurate and reduce childhood mortality. Health workers in the field send a child's age, height, and weight by SMS to a central server, which determines whether the child is at risk and sends a message back to the health worker.

The use of the existing technology infrastructure would be useful in any part of the world where health care resources are scarce. Yet this approach can also provide benefits in developed countries. Technology could be used, for example, to reduce emergency-room overcrowding by providing phone- or Internet-based advice and triage services during evenings and weekends. Similarly, it could be used to deliver care remotely for patients who require ongoing treatment for diabetes, asthma, or other chronic diseases.

'RIGHT SKILL' THE WORKFORCE

Some smart innovators challenge existing practices—and professional assumptions—about which health workers are allowed to do what. As a result, they can tightly link skills and training requirements to the tasks at hand, thereby lowering labour costs and overcoming labour constraints. In India, LifeSpring uses midwives to provide most of the care at its maternity hospitals. This allows just a single doctor to oversee significantly more patients by focusing on tasks that specifically require a doctor's attention. The company charges only $40 for a normal delivery, rather than the typical $200. In the United States, MinuteClinic uses nurse-practitioners rather than physicians to staff primary-care clinics.

In some countries, this approach also helps to ameliorate shortages of medical talent. In sub-Saharan Africa, for example, the HealthStore Foundation has trained community health workers to diagnose and treat the region's top five diseases, which together account for more than half of preventable deaths there.

STANDARDIZE OPERATING PROCEDURES

Whenever possible, successful innovators use highly standardized operating procedures to minimize waste and improve the utilization of labour and assets. The use of standardized clinical protocols also raises the quality of care and facilitates the transfer of knowledge. In India, Aravind Eye Care System, which provides cataract operations to the blind and the near-blind, standardizes the entire end-to-end patient pathway—from initial diagnosis to surgery, recovery, and discharge—with ruthless efficiency.

Also in India, Narayana Hrudayalaya hospitals can offer high-quality cardiac care at dramatically lower prices than its competitors charge because it employs a high-volume, highly standardized model of care. Both organizations use a form of production specialization (a factory-like approach to delivering care), borrowing process flow, management, and improvement techniques from manufacturing industries.

BORROW SOMEONE ELSE'S ASSETS

Smart innovators use existing institutions, infrastructure, and networks of people to reduce capital investments and operating costs. They then pass the savings on to consumers. India's Health Management Research Institute (HMRI) takes advantage of established supply chains by operating medical convoys—mobile health facilities and health workers delivering care in hard- to-reach rural areas—from public hospitals.

HMRI also operates a medical hotline (dial 104 for 24/7 advice) that piggybacks on existing mobile-phone systems, as do MedicallHome, Pesinet, and similar organizations. The model benefits from the widespread adoption of mobile phones and a comprehensive cell network across India. MinuteClinic operates its facilities in retail stores to benefit from their foot traffic and lower its overhead costs.

OPEN UP NEW REVENUE STREAMS

Many health care innovators extend their activities into other sectors—even shops and restaurants—to capture additional revenue streams, use them to subsidize costs, or both. Business activities in other sectors can even promote core health care services. Thailand's Population and Community Development Association (PDA), which focuses on family planning and the prevention of sexually transmitted diseases, established a chain of restaurants and resorts to raise revenue—and to get out the message. Greenstar, a Pakistani non- governmental organization that focuses on family planning, operates an entire network of retail outlets that sell products such as condoms and offer family- planning advice and health services for women and children.

MARKETING CONCEPT IN HEALTH-CARE SERVICES

Health-care services represent the biggest and fastest growing segment of the United States' economy. For some perspective, the U.S. spends about double that of other advanced nations as a share of GDP (>10%) (Conrad, 2009) Nevertheless, our system is in a serious financial crisis and "expected to get worse as the population ages and costs continue to rise."(Carter, 2007) The current health-care debate related to marketplace reform is only one outgrowth (i.e. who will be covered and how will that coverage be subsidized?).

Contributing to the larger crisis is the ever-changing marketplace, from rapidly advancing technology and medical science with its corresponding new treatment options, to the persistent erosion of the tertiary–level hospital, to changing demography (aging "Boomers").

These and other shifts have affected virtually every area of health-care delivery. The increasing stressors will continue to challenge marketing planners and decision-makers who interface directly with patients as service providers, as never before.

The purpose of this chapter is to share the experience of one hospital's efforts to enhance their marketing performance through their continuing efforts to monitor their patient service area and deliver value consistent with their continuing consumer-oriented research programme (i.e. implementation of the marketing concept).

HOSPITAL MARKET PLANNING

Market planning in general refers to considering those marketing activities which serve to identify and help develop specific courses of action necessary to achieve future marketing goals. In terms of hospital market planning, a variety of organizational goals have traditionally been involved such as achievement of a specific and/or stable census, or achieving prescribed benchmarks on various financial metrics such as a specific ROI, or achieving external recognitions resulting from performance effectiveness and associated rankings.

The problems with these types of goals is that they (1) tend to de-value the role of individual patients and their impact on marketing-related goals (e.g. patient satisfaction (CRM), long-term patient loyalty (LTV), capturing new and opportune market positions, and various promotional outcomes such as name recognition, awareness of basic services, and points of distinction, etc., and (2) they have given rise to the view of a highly fragmented health care marketplace.

For instance, among the competing "markets" typically associated with hospital performance in addition to patients themselves, are physicians, community agencies, regulatory bodies from various levels of government, third-party payers, philanthropists, and institutional suppliers, and even Boards of Trustees. Unfortunately, current evidence supports the conclusion that while more health care providers talk about the patient market as the most important primary objective, few actively measure their success through patient satisfaction.

THE MARKETING CONCEPT

Simply put, the marketing concept is the most widely endorsed, contemporary philosophy for practicing marketing. As defined in most marketing texts, the basic notion is that an organization will best achieve long- term marketing goals through an awareness of the specific wants and needs of the parties with whom it exchanges value, and a dedication of the entire organization's efforts towards fulfilling those wants and needs better than competitors. Every opportunity for exchange must be carefully analyzed, understood, and managed to ensure each party's maximum satisfaction. Integrated marketing is typically used to describe the primary organizational challenge of the marketing concept that every member of the organization, from the CEO to the custodial staff must be authorized and expected to deliver maximum satisfaction to meet specific needs in the right way, at the right price, in the right location. Wherever and whenever the need arises relevant to the organization's mission, the organization must be prepared and equipped to turn the unmet need into a satisfying exchange of value for their customer(s) and thereby achieve their own organizational goals. Research has shown in general that a "one percent increase in satisfaction can produce up to a three percent increase in capitalization" (Friar, 2001). Further, as health care providers rely more heavily on serving patient's expectations, the chances of achieving patient satisfaction also increases (Bedi, et al, 2004).

PATIENT SERVICE AREA

Brottman Hospital is located in a relatively insulated city with a population of approximately 100,000. It is one of three, roughly equal-sized tertiary hospitals in the city which have competed against one another for several years. Each is geographically located essentially equidistant from one another and each has access to approximately equal population densities within its immediate patient service areas. Thus, among their competitive advantages, each claimed a geographic portion of the city as their own by virtue of their locations. Administrators at all three typically viewed this separation as their competitive fait accompli, and their primary market areas were fairly stable and rarely challenged. The typical operating assumptions and often the primary impetus to market planning was the need/ability to successfully retain their respective fair-share, one-third of the city-wide demand for hospital services. The competitive atmosphere was often characterized as cooperative. Correspondingly, marketing planning activities at Brottman often appeared half-hearted and generally unimportant.

THE SHAKE-UP

Despite the rather benign and harmonious competitive environment and apathy towards planning, administrators at Brottman had nonetheless retained the services of a marketing research consulting firm for many years. The firm was charged with delivering an annual report on community-wide attitudes, opinions, and beliefs about the entire patient service area. From an outsider's perspective, it appeared to serve more as a report-card than a basis for diagnosing key opportunities or threats. Every year, a telephone survey of 400-500 randomly-selected households with numbers listed in the local phone directory was conducted resulting in usable samples generally ranging between 300-350 usable responses. All respondents were asked to confirm their addresses with the local directory. The questionnaire was suitable for telephone delivery and asked several qualifying questions about each hospital.

Brottman was never disclosed as the sponsor. Profiles of city resident's opinions and general attitudes of the hospitals were compiled and compared longitudinally to previous studies. These profiles were then distributed to key administrators, discussed in administrative meetings, and portions were shared with employees through formal departmental meetings. But as the role of the marketing concept in health care and hospital services grew in popularity and more research highlighted the potential of marketing activities to improve the performance of the health care industry, administrators at Brottman began to turn their attention towards their delivery of emergency services.

The nearest trauma center was over 70 miles away, and none of the three local hospitals was fully equipped to handle extensive, critical trauma, services. In addition, Brottman increasingly recognized the E-R as a gateway for those all important institutional first-impressions and the foundation for a lifetime of health care delivery opportunities. They had long been aware that proximity to an E-R was the foremost decision factor for most patients in a time of need.

Coincidentally, at about this same time, a major-name hospital from a neighbouring, but larger city, announced plans to develop a satellite, convenient and emergi-care clinic in the city. The long-held assumption that proximity provided sanctuary, was about to be challenged as never before. Thus, quickly rising on the list of their developing research priorities was the need to identify consumer preferences for all the city's emergency rooms, and to more fully assess the potential of the E-R to provide competitive advantage against the invaders.

MARKET PLANNING

Among the many models available to aid in the diagnosis and measurement of impact of changes in key marketing parameters, Markov analysis (MA) has proven useful in a variety of applications (Garg & McClean, 2009; Bala & Mauskopf, 2006; Barton, et al 2004; Portela & Simpson, 1996). It has its roots in basic probability theory and has been useful for projecting the effect or impact of present policies on future market positions. By extrapolating current market shares through the use of transition probabilities, estimates (or simulations) of equilibrium market shares can be generated.If a firm were to determine that its future market share was jeopardized by changing consumer preferences, it could conceivably take counter-measures to correct the undesirable trend. Similarly, if the opposite were true, it could engage reinforcing activity to enhance favourable trends. MA not only has the potential to assist in the identification of tomorrow's outcomes from today's marketing actions/ inactions, but it also has the advantage of resembling the basic tenets of unit analysis (Cravens, 1982), or the disaggregation of competitive data for planning purposes.

Since these units might generally represent distinctive sets of products, market segments, or organizational centers, the changing E-R situation at Brottman seemed well suited for a test of its applicability. Both the long-term assumptions about the stability of three hospital's market shares as well as the impending and dramatic competitive intrusion, added further appeal for its application.

Two elements of the survey instrument which presented the opportunity to apply MA were (1) a measure of the physical proximity of each respondent to their nearest E-R, and (2) a measures of each respondent's preference for an E-R in the city, in the event an emergency situation occurred. Each respondent's residence was identified on a city map and the distance to the nearest hospital was determined based on straight-line measures. There were a few cases where respondents were located equidistant from two hospitals and they were omitted from this study.

MARKETS AND FINANCE IN HEALTH CARE

Health care spending in the United States is characterized as being the most costly per person as compared to all other countries, and despite this spending, the quality of health care overall is low by some measures.

The Centers for Medicare and Medicaid reported in 2013 that U.S. health care costs were 17.9% GDP in 2011, similar to 2010 and 2009 but up from 13.8% GDP in 2000. Health care costs per capita have risen steadily from $4,878 in 2000 to $8,680 in 2011, a 5.4% average annual increase. The annual rate of increase in total health care costs has been declining, falling steadily from a 9.7% increase in 2002 to 3.9% for 2009, 2010 and 2011.

The Congressional Budget Office reported in February 2013 that Medicare costs were 3.5% GDP in 2012, down from 3.7% GDP in 2011 but up from 2.2% GDP in 2000. Medicaid costs were 1.6% GDP in 2012, down from 1.8% GDP in 2011 but up from 1.2% GDP in 2000. CBO projected in June 2012 that federal spending on health care programmes will rise from 5.4% GDP in 2012 to 9.6% GDP by 2037. This would be driven by a significant increase in the number of programme beneficiaries due to the retirement of the Baby Boomers, along with health care cost inflation.

According to the World Health Organization (WHO), total health care spending in the U.S. was 15.2% of itsGDP in 2008, the highest in the world. The Health and Human Services Department expects that the health share of GDP will continue its historical upward trend, reaching 19.5% of GDP by 2017. Of each dollar spent on health care in the United States, 31% goes to hospital care, 21% goes to physician/clinical services, 10% to pharmaceuticals, 4% to dental, 6% to nursing homes and 3% to home health care, 3% for other retail products, 3% for government public health activities, 7% to administrative costs, 7% toinvestment, and 6% to other professional services (physical therapists, optometrists, etc.). TheCommonwealth Fund ranked the United States last in the quality of health care among similar countries,and notes U.S. care costs the most.

Around 84.7% of Americans have some form of health insurance; either through their employer or the employer of their spouse or parent (59.3%), purchased individually (8.9%), or provided by government programmes (27.8%; there is some overlap in these figures). All government health care programmes have restricted eligibility, and there is no government health insurance company which covers all Americans. Americans without health insurance coverage in 2007 totaled 15.3% of the population, or 45.7 million people.Among those whose employer pays for health insurance, the employee may be required to contribute part of the cost of this insurance, while the employer usually chooses the insurance company and, for large groups, negotiates with the insurance company. Government programmes directly cover 27.8% of the population (83 million), including the elderly, disabled, children, veterans, and some of the poor, and federal law mandates public access to emergency services regardless of ability to pay. Public spending accounts for between 45% and 56.1% of U.S. health care spending.

Some Americans do not qualify for government-provided health insurance, are not provided health insurance by an employer, and are unable to afford, cannot qualify for, or choose not to purchase, private health insurance. When charity or "uncompensated" care is not available, they sometimes simply go without needed medical treatment. This problem has become a source of considerable political controversy on a national level.

SPENDING

PER CAPITA

The Office of the Actuary (OACT) of the Centers for Medicare and Medicaid Services publishes data on total health care spending in the United States, including both historical levels and future projections. In 2007, the U.S. spent $2.26 trillion on health care, or $7,439 per person, up from $2.1 trillion, or $7,026 per capita, the previous year. Spending in 2006 represented 16% of GDP, an increase of 6.7% over 2004 spending. Growth in spending is projected to average 6.7% annually over the period 2007 through 2017. In 2009, the United States federal, state and local governments, corporations and individuals, together spent $2.5 trillion, $8,047 per person, on health care. This amount represented 17.3% of the GDP, up from 16.2% in 2008. Health insurance costs are rising faster than wages or inflation, and medical causes were cited by about half of bankruptcy filers in the United States in 2001.

RATE OF INCREASE

The Centers for Medicare and Medicaid Services reported in 2013 that the rate of increase in annual health care costs has fallen since 2002. However, costs relative to GDP and per capita continue to rise. Per capita cost increases have averaged 5.4% since 2000.

Several studies have attempted to explain the reduction in the rate of annual increase. Reasons include, among others:

- Higher unemployment due to the 2008-2012 recession, which has limited the ability of consumers to purchase health care;
- Rising out-of-pocket payments;
- Deductibles (the amount a person pays before insurance begins to cover claims) have risen sharply. Workers must pay a larger share of their own health costs, and generally forces them to spend less; and.

- The proportion of workers with employer-sponsored health insurance enrolled in a plan that required a deductible climbed to about three-quarters in 2012 from about half in 2006.

In September 2008 The Wall Street Journal reported that consumers were reducing their health care spending in response to the current economic slow-down. Both the number of prescriptions filled and the number of office visits dropped between 2007 and 2008. In one survey, 22% of consumers reported going to the doctor less often, and 11% reported buying fewer prescription drugs.

RELATIVE TO OTHER COUNTRIES

One analysis of international spending levels in the year 2000 found that while the U.S. spends more on health care than other countries in the Organisation for Economic Co-operation and Development (OECD), the use of health care services in the U.S. is below the OECD median by most measures. The authors of the study concluded that the prices paid for health care services are much higher in the U.S. Economist Hans Sennholz has argued that the Medicare and Medicaid programmes may be the main reason for rising health care costs in the U.S.

CONCENTRATION

Health care spending in the United States is concentrated. An analysis of the 2008 and 2009 data by Agency for Health care Research and Quality (AHRQ) found that the 1% of the population with the highest spending accounted for 27% of aggregate health care spending.

The highest-spending 5% of the population accounted for more than half of all spending. This reflects spending in 2009, as well. In both 2008 and 2009, the top 30 percent of the population ranked by expenditures accounted for nearly 89 percent of health care expenditures. Further, the bottom 50 percent of the population ranked by their expenditures accounted for only 3.1 percent and 2.9 percent of the total for 2008 and 2009.

Relative to the overall population, those who remained in the top 10% of spenders between 2008 and 2009 were more likely to be in fair or poor health, elderly, female, non-Hispanic whites and those with public-only coverage. Those who remained in the bottom half of spenders were more likely to be in excellent health, children and young adults, men, Hispanics, and the uninsured. These patterns were stable through the 1970s and 1980s, and some data suggest that they may have been typical of the mid-to-early 20th century as well.

An earlier study by AHRQ the found significant persistence in the level of health care spending from year to year. Of the 1% of the population with the highest health care spending in 2002, 24.3% maintained their ranking in the top 1% in 2003. Of the 5% with the highest spending in 2002, 34% maintained that ranking in 2003. Individuals over age 45 were disproportionately represented among those who were in the top decile of spending for both years.

Seniors spend, on average, far more on health care costs than either working-age adults or children. The pattern of spending by age was stable for most ages from 1987 through 2004, with the exception of spending for seniors age 85 and over. Spending for this group grew less rapidly than that of other groups over this period.

The 2008 edition of the Dartmouth Atlas of Health Care found that providing Medicare beneficiaries with severe chronic illnesses with more intense health care in the last two years of life—increased spending, more tests, more procedures and longer hospital stays—is not associated with better patient outcomes. There are significant geographic variations in the level of care provided to chronically ill patients, only 4% of which are explained by differences in the number of severely ill people in an area. Most of the differences are explained by differences in the amount of "supply-sensitive" care available in an area. Acute hospital care accounts for over half (55%) of the spending for Medicare beneficiaries in the last two years of life, and differences in the volume of services provided is more significant than differences in price. The researchers found no evidence of "substitution" of care, where increased use of hospital care would reduce outpatient spending (or vice versa).

HOSPITALIZATION COSTS

According to a report from the Agency for Health care Research and Quality (AHRQ), aggregate U.S. hospital costs in 2011 were $387.3 billion—a 63% increase since 1997 (inflation adjusted). Costs per stay increased 47% since 1997, averaging $10,000 in 2011.

CBO ANALYSIS

The Congressional Budget Office reported in February 2013 that Medicare costs were 3.5% GDP in 2012, down from 3.7% GDP in 2011 but up from 2.2% GDP in 2000. Medicaid costs were 1.6% GDP in 2012, down from 1.8% GDP in 2011 but up from 1.2% GDP in 2000.

CBO projected in June 2012 that federal spending on health care programmes will rise from 5.4% GDP in 2012 to 9.6% GDP by 2037. This would be driven by a significant increase in the number of programme beneficiaries due to the retirement of the Baby Boomers, along with health care cost inflation.

PRIVATE

Most Americans under age 65 (59.3%) receive their health insurance coverage through an employer (which includes both private as well as civilian public-sector employers) under group coverage, although this percentage is declining. Costs for employer-paid health insurance are rising rapidly: since 2001, premiums for family coverage have increased 78%, while wages have risen 19% and inflation has risen 17%, according to a 2007 study by the Kaiser Family Foundation.

Workers with employer-sponsored insurance also contribute; in 2007, the average percentage of premium paid by covered workers is 16% for single coverage and 28% for family coverage. In addition to their premium contributions, most covered workers face additional payments when they use health care services, in the form of deductibles and copayments.

Just less than 9% of the population purchases individual health care insurance. Insurance payments are a form of cost-sharing and risk management where each individual or their employer pays predictable monthly premiums. This cost-spreading mechanism often picks up much of the cost of health care, but individuals must often pay up-front a minimum part of the total cost (a deductible), or a small part of the cost of every procedure (a copayment). Private insurance accounts for 35% of total health spending in the United States, by far the largest share among OECD countries. Beside the United States, Canada and France are the two other OECD countries where private insurance represents more than 10% of total health spending.

Provider networks can be used to reduce costs by negotiating favourable fees from providers, selecting cost effective providers, and creating financial incentives for providers to practice more efficiently. A survey issued in 2009 by America's Health Insurance Plans found that patients going to out-of- network providers are sometimes charged extremely high fees. Defying many analysts' expectations, PPOs have gained market share at the expense of HMOs over the past decade.

Just as the more loosely managed PPOs have edged out HMOs, HMOs themselves have also evolved towards less tightly managed models. The first HMOs in the U.S., such as Kaiser Permanente in Oakland, California, and the Health Insurance Plan (HIP) in New York, were "staff-model" HMOs, which owned their own health care facilities and employed the doctors and other health care professionals who staffed them. The name health maintenance organization stems from the idea that the HMO would make it its job to maintain the enrollee's health, rather than merely to treat illnesses. In accordance with this mission, managed care organizations typically cover preventive health care. Within the tightly integrated staff-model HMO, the HMO can develop and disseminate guidelines on cost-effective care, while the enrollee's primary care doctor can act as patient advocate and care coordinator, helping the patient negotiate the complex health care system.

Despite a substantial body of research demonstrating that many staff- model HMOs deliver high-quality and cost-effective care, they have steadily lost market share. They have been replaced by more loosely managed networks of providers with whom health plans have negotiated discounted fees. It is common today for a physician or hospital to have contracts with a dozen or more health plans, each with different referral networks, contracts with different diagnostic facilities, and different practice guidelines.

PUBLIC

Government programmes directly cover 27.8% of the population (83 million), including the elderly, disabled, children, veterans, and some of the poor, and federal law mandates public access to emergency services regardless of ability to pay. Public spending accounts for between 45% and 56.1% of U.S. health care spending. Per-capita spending on health care by the U.S. government placed it among the top ten highest spenders among United Nations member countries in 2004.

However, all government-funded health care programmes exist only in the form of statutory law, and accordingly can be amended or revoked like any other statute. There is no constitutional right to health care. The U.S.

Supreme Court explained in 1977 that "the Constitution imposes no obligation on the States to pay ... any of the medical expenses of indigents."

Government funded programmes include:

- National Institutes of Health treats patients who enroll in research for free.
- Medical Corps of various branches of the military.
- Certain county and state hospitals.
- Government run community clinics.

The exemption of employer-sponsored health benefits from federal income and payroll taxes distorts the health care market. The U.S. government, unlike some other countries, does not treat employer funded health care benefits as a taxable benefit in kind to the employee. The value of the lost tax revenue from a benefits in kind tax is an estimated $150 billion a year. Some regard this as being disadvantageous to people who have to buy insurance in the individual market which must be paid from income received after tax. Health insurance benefits are an attractive way for employers to increase the salary of employees as they are non-taxable.

As a result, 65% of the non-elderly population and over 90% of the privately insured non-elderly population receives health insurance at the workplace. Additionally, most economists agree that this tax shelter increases individual demand for health insurance, leading some to claim that it is largely responsible for the rise in health care spending.

In addition the government allows full tax shelter at the highest marginal rate to investors in health savings accounts (HSAs). Some have argued that this tax incentive adds little value to national health care as a whole because the most wealthy in society tend also to be the most healthy. Also it has been argued, HSAs segregate the insurance pools into those for the wealthy and those for the less wealthy which thereby makes equivalent insurance cheaper for the rich and more expensive for the poor. However, one advantage of health insurance accounts is that funds can only be used towards certain HSA qualified expenses, including medicine, doctor's fees, and Medicare Parts A and B. Funds cannot be used towards expenses such as cosmetic surgery.

There are also various state and local programmes for the poor. In 2007, Medicaid provided health care coverage for 39.6 million low-income Americans (although Medicaid covers approximately 40% of America's poor), and Medicare provided health care coverage for 41.4 million elderly and disabled Americans. Enrollment in Medicare is expected to reach 77 million by 2031, when the baby boom generation is fully enrolled.

It has been reported that the number of physicians accepting Medicaid has decreased in recent years due to relatively high administrative costs and low reimbursements. In 1997, the federal government also created the State Children's Health Insurance Programme (SCHIP), a joint federal-state programme to insure children in families that earn too much to qualify for Medicaid but cannot afford health insurance. SCHIP covered 6.6 million children in 2006,but the programme is already facing funding shortfalls in many states. The government has also mandated access to emergency care regardless of insurance status and ability to pay through the Emergency Medical Treatment and Labour Act (EMTALA), passed in 1986, but EMTALA is an unfunded mandate.

THE UNINSURED

NUMBER OF UNINSURED

Some Americans do not qualify for government-provided health insurance, are not provided health insurance by an employer, and are unable to afford, cannot qualify for, or choose not to purchase, private health insurance. When charity or "uncompensated" care is not available, they sometimes simply go without needed medical treatment. This problem has become a source of considerable political controversy on a national level.

According to the US Census Bureau, in 2007, 45.7 million people in the U.S. (15.3% of the population) were without health insurance for at least part of the year. This number was down slightly from the previous year, with nearly 3 million more people receiving government coverage and a slightly lower percentage covered under private plans than the year previous. Other studies have placed the number of uninsured in the years 2007–2008 as high as 86.7 million, about 29% of the US population.

Among the uninsured population, the Census Bureau says, nearly 37 million were employment-age adults (ages 18 to 64), and more than 27 million worked at least part-time. About 38% of the uninsured live in households with incomes of $50,000 or more. According to the Census Bureau, nearly 36 million of the uninsured are legal U.S citizens. Another 9.7 million are non- citizens, but the Census Bureau does not distinguish in its estimate between legal non-citizens and illegal immigrants. Nearly one fifth of the uninsured population is able to afford insurance, almost one quarter is eligible for public coverage, and the remaining 56% need financial assistance (8.9% of all Americans). Extending coverage to all who are eligible remains a fiscal challenge.

A 2003 study in Health Affairs estimated that uninsured people in the U.S. received approximately $35 billion in uncompensated care in 2001. The study noted that this amount per capita was half what the average insured person received. The study found that various levels of government finance most uncompensated care, spending about $30.6 billion on payments and programmes to serve the uninsured and covering as much as 80–85% of uncompensated care costs through grants and other direct payments, tax appropriations, and Medicare and Medicaid payment add-ons. Most of this money comes from the federal government, followed by state and local tax appropriations for hospitals. Another study by the same authors in the same year estimated the additional annual cost of covering the uninsured (in 2001 dollars) at $34 billion (for public coverage) and $69 billion (for private coverage).

These estimates represent an increase in total health care spending of 3–6% and would raise health care's share of GDP by less than one percentage point, the study concluded. Another study published in the same journal in 2004 estimated that the value of health forgone each year because of uninsurance was $65–$130 billion and concluded that this figure constituted "a lower-bound estimate of economic losses resulting from the present level of uninsurance nationally."

The health insurance system in America, in contrast with health insurance in almost all other developed nations, is fundamentally a voluntary one. There are many perspectives on the purpose of health insurance in the United States. For consumers, health insurance serves two main purposes: it provides access to affordable health care through preferential pricing and it offers financial protection from unexpected health care costs. For clinicians and other health care providers, insurance ensures financial stability of the practice/office. Health insurance was first developed by Baylor University Hospital for exactly that purpose.

EFFECTS ON UNINSURED

From 2000 to 2004, the Institute of Medicine's Committee on the Consequences of Uninsurance issued a series of six reports that reviewed and reported on the evidence on the effects of the lack of health insurance coverage.

The reports concluded that the committee recommended that the nation should implement a strategy to achieve universal health insurance coverage. As of 2011, a comprehensive national plan to address what universal health plan supporters terms "America's uninsured crisis", has yet to be enacted. A few states have achieved progress towards the goal of universal health insurance coverage, such as Maine, Massachusetts, and Vermont, but other states including California, have failed attempts of reforms.

The six reports created by the Institute of Medicine (IOM) found that the principal consequences of uninsurance were the following: Children and Adults without health insurance did not receive needed medical care; they typically live in poorer health and die earlier than children or adults who have insurance. The financial stability of a whole family can be put at risk if only one person is uninsured and needs treatment for unexpected health care costs. The overall health status of a community can be adversely affected by a higher percentage of uninsured people within the community. The coverage gap between the insured and the uninsured has not decreased even after the recent federal initiatives to extend health insurance coverage.

The last report was published in 2004 and was named Insuring America's Health: Principles and Recommendations. This report recommended the following: The President and Congress need to develop a strategy to achieve universal insurance coverage and establish a firm schedule to reach this goal by the year 2010. The committee also recommended that the federal and state governments provide sufficient resources for Medicaid and the State Children's Health Insurance Programme (SCHIP) to cover all persons currently eligible until the universal coverage takes effect. They also warned that the federal and state governments should prevent the erosion of outreach efforts, eligibility, enrollment, and coverage of these specific programmes.

Some people think that not having health insurance will have adverse consequences for the health of the uninsured. On the other hand, some people believe that children and adults without health insurance have access to needed health care services at hospital emergency rooms, community health centers, or other safety net facilities offering charity care. Some observers note that there is a solid body of evidence showing that a substantial proportion of U.S. health care expenditures is directed towards care that is not effective and may sometimes even be harmful. At least for the insured population, spending more and using more health care services does not always yield better health outcomes or increase life expectancy.

Children in America are typically perceived as in good health relative to adults, due to the fact that most serious health problems occur later in one's life. Certain conditions including asthma, diabetes, and obesity have become much more prevalent among children in the past few decades. There is also a growing population of vulnerable children with special health care needs that require ongoing medical attention, which would not be accessible without health insurance. More than 10 million children in the United States meet the federal definition of children with special health care needs "who have or are at increased risk for a chronic physical, development, behavioral, or emotional condition and who also require health and related services of a type or amount beyond that required by children generally".

These children require health related services of an amount beyond that required by the average children in America. Typically when children acquire health insurance, they are much less likely to experience previously unmet health care needs, this includes the average child in America and children with special health care needs. The Committee on Health Insurance Status and Its Consequences concluded that the effects of health insurance on children's health outcomes: Children with health insurance receive more timely diagnosis of serious health conditions, experience fewer hospitalizations, and miss fewer days of school.

The same committee analyzed the effects of health insurance on adult's health outcomes: adults who do not have health insurance coverage who acquire Medicare coverage at age 65, experience substantially improved health and functional status, particularly those who have cardiovascular disease or diabetes. Adults who have cardiovascular disease or other cardiac risk factors that are uninsured are less likely to be aware of their condition, which leads to worse health outcomes for those individuals.

Without health insurance, adults are more likely to be diagnosed with certain cancers that would have been detectable earlier by screening by a clinician if they had regularly visited a doctor. As a consequence, these adults are more likely to die from their diagnosed cancer or suffer poorer health outcomes.

Many towns and cities in the United States have high concentrations of people under the age of 65 who lack health insurance. There are implications of high rates of uninsurance for communities and for insured people in those communities. Institute of Medicine committee warned of the potential problems of high rates of uninsurance for local health care, including reduced access to clinic-based primary care, specialty services, and hospital-based emergency services.

EXPENDITURES BY THE UNINSURED

Estimates for 2008 reported that the uninsured would spend $30 billion for health care and receive $56 billion in uncompensated care, and that if everyone were covered by insurance then overall costs would increase by $123 billion. A 2003 Institute of Medicine (IOM) report estimated total cost of health in out-of-pocket spending by the uninsured, with $34.5 billion in "free" "uncompensated" care covered by government subsidies of $30.6 billion to hospitals and clinics and $5.1 billion in donated services by physicians.

ROLE OF GOVERNMENT IN HEALTH CARE MARKET

Numerous publicly funded health care programmes help to provide for the elderly, disabled, military service families and veterans, children, and the poor,and federal law ensures public access to emergency services regardless of ability to pay; however, a system of universal health care has not been implemented nation-wide. However, as the OECD has pointed out, the total U.S. public expenditure for this limited population would, in most other OECD countries, be enough for the government to provide primary health insurance for the entire population.

Although the federal Medicare programme and the federal-state Medicaid programmes possess some monopsonistic purchasing power, the highly fragmented buy side of the U.S. health system is relatively weak by international standards, and in some areas, some suppliers such as large hospital groups have a virtual monopoly on the supply side. In most OECD countries, there is a high degree of public ownership and public finance. The resulting economy of scale in providing health care services appears to enable a much tighter grip on costs. The U.S., as a matter of oft-stated public policy, largely does not regulate prices of services from private providers, assuming the private sector to do it better.

Massachusetts has adopted a universal health care system through the Massachusetts 2006 Health Reform Statute. It mandates that all residents who can afford to do so purchase health insurance, provides subsidized insurance plans so that nearly everyone can afford health insurance, and provides a "Health Safety Net Fund" to pay for necessary treatment for those who cannot find affordable health insurance or are not eligible. In July 2009, Connecticut passed into law a plan called SustiNet, with the goal of achieving health-care coverage of 98% of its residents by 2014.

IMPACT ON U.S. ECONOMIC PRODUCTIVITY

On March 1, 2010, billionaire investor Warren Buffett said that the high costs paid by U.S. companies for their employees' health care put them at a competitive disadvantage. He compared the roughly 17% of GDP spent by the U.S. on health care with the 9% of GDP spent by much of the rest of the world, noted that the U.S. has fewer doctors and nurses per person, and said, "[t]hat kind of a cost, compared with the rest of the world, is like a tapeworm eating at our economic body."

PROPOSED SOLUTIONS

Increased spending on disease prevention is often suggested as a way of reducing health care spending. Whether prevention saves or costs money depends on the intervention. Childhood vaccinations, or contraceptives save much more than they cost. Research suggests that in many cases prevention does not produce significant long-term cost savings.

Some interventions may be cost-effective by providing health benefits, while others are not cost-effective. Preventive care is typically provided to many people who would never become ill, and for those who would have become ill is partially offset by the health care costs during additional years of life. On the other hand, research conducted by Novartis argues that the countries that have excelled in getting the highest value for health care spending are the ones who have invested more in prevention, early diagnosis and treatment. The trick is to avoid getting patients to hospital, which is where highest health care dollars are being consumed.

Not all preventive measures have good ROI (EG. Global vaccination campaign for a rare infectious diseases). However, preventive measures such as diet, exercises and reduction of tobacco intake would have broad impact on many diseases and will offer good return of investment.

Eliminating waste is another solution. In December 2011, the outgoing Administrator of the Centers for Medicare & Medicaid Services, Dr. Donald Berwick, asserted that 20% to 30% of health care spending is waste. He listed five causes for the waste: (1) overtreatment of patients, (2) the failure to coordinate care, (3) the administrative complexity of the health care system, (4) burdensome rules and (5) fraud.

FINANCIAL RESOURCES

There are generally five primary methods of funding health systems:

1. General taxation to the state, county or municipality.
2. Social health insurance.
3. Voluntary or private health insurance.
4. Out-of-pocket payments.
5. Donations to charities.

Most countries' systems feature a mix of all five models. One study based on data from the OECD concluded that all types of health care finance "are compatible with" an efficient health system. The study also found no relationship between financing and cost control.

The term health insurance is generally used to describe a form of insurance that pays for medical expenses. It is sometimes used more broadly to include insurance covering disability or long-term nursing or custodial careneeds. It may be provided through a social insurance programme, or from private insurance companies. It may be obtained on a group basis (e.g., by a firm to cover its employees) or purchased by individual consumers. In each case premiums or taxes protect the insured from high or unexpected health care expenses.

By estimating the overall cost of health care expenses, a routine finance structure (such as a monthly premium or annual tax) can be developed, ensuring that money is available to pay for the health care benefits specified in the insurance agreement. The benefit is typically administered by a government agency, a non-profit health fund or a corporation operating seeking to make a profit.

Many forms of commercial health insurance control their costs by restricting the benefits that are paid by through deductibles, co-payments, coinsurance, policy exclusions, and total coverage limits and will severely restrict or refuse coverage of pre-existing conditions. Many government schemes also have co-payment schemes but exclusions are rare because of political pressure. The larger insurance schemes may also negotiate fees with providers.

Many forms of social insurance schemes control their costs by using the bargaining power of their community they represent to control costs in the health care delivery system. For example by negotiating drug prices directly with pharmaceutical companies, or negotiating standard fees with the medical profession. Social schemes sometimes feature contributions related to earnings as part of a scheme to deliver universal health care, which may or may not also involve the use of commercial and non-commercial insurers. Essentially the more wealthy pay proportionately more into the scheme to cover the needs of the relatively poor who therefore contribute proportionately less.

There are usually caps on the contributions of the wealthy and minimum payments that must be made by the insured (often in the form of a minimum contribution, similar to a deductible in commercial insurance models).

In addition to these traditional health care financing methods, some lower income countries and development partners are also implementing non- traditional or innovative financing mechanisms for scaling up delivery and sustainability of health care, such as micro-contributions, public-private partnerships, and market-based financial transaction taxes. For example, as of June 2011, UNITAID had collected more than one billion dollars from 29 member countries, including several from Africa, through an air ticket solidarity levy to expand access to care and treatment for HIV/ AIDS, tuberculosis and malaria in 94 countries.

PAYMENT MODELS

In most countries, wage costs for health care practitioners are estimated to represent between 65% and 80% of renewable health system expenditures.

There are three ways to pay medical practitioners: fee for service, capitation, and salary. There has been growing interest in blending elements of these systems.

FEE-FOR-SERVICE

Fee-for-service arrangements pay general practitioners (GPs) based on the service. They are even more widely used for specialists working inambulatory care.

There are two ways to set fee levels:

- By individual practitioners.
- Central negotiations (as in Japan, Germany, Canada and in France) or hybrid model (such as in Australia, France's sector 2, and New Zealand) where GPs can charge extra fees on top of standardized patient reimbursement rates.

CAPITATION

In capitation payment systems, GPs are paid for each patient on their "list", usually with adjustments for factors such as age and gender. According to OECD, "these systems are used in Italy (with some fees), in all four countries of the United Kingdom (with some fees and allowances for specific services), Austria (with fees for specific services), Denmark (one third of income with remainder fee for service), Ireland (since 1989), the Netherlands (fee-for-service for privately insured patients and public employees) and Sweden (from 1994). Capitation payments have become more frequent in "managed care" environments in the United States."

According to OECD, "Capitation systems allow funders to control the overall level of primary health expenditures, and the allocation of funding among GPs is determined by patient registrations. However, under this approach, GPs may register too many patients and under- serve them, select the better risks and refer on patients who could have been treated by the GP directly.

Freedom of consumer choice over doctors, coupled with the principle of "money following the patient" may moderate some of these risks. Aside from selection, these problems are likely to be less marked than under salary-type arrangements."

SALARY ARRANGEMENTS

In several OECD countries, general practitioners (GPs) are employed on salaries for the government. According to OECD, "Salary arrangements allow funders to control primary care costs directly; however, they may lead to under- provision of services (to ease workloads), excessive referrals to secondary providers and lack of attention to the preferences of patients." There has been movement away from this system.

MARKETING DEMAND FOR HEALTH CARE

The demand for health care is a derived demand from the supply for health. Health care is demanded as a means for consumers to achieve a larger stock of "health capital." The demand for health is unlike most other goods because individuals allocate resources in order to both consume and produce health. The description gives three roles of persons in health economics.

The World Health Report states that people take four roles in the health care:

1. Contributors
2. Citizens
3. Providers
4. Consumers

Michael Grossman's 1972 model of health production has been extremely influential in this field of study and has several unique elements that make it notable. Grossman's model views each individual as both a producer and a consumer of health. Health is treated as a stock which degrades over time in the absence of "investments" in health, so that health is viewed as a sort of capital.

The model acknowledges that health is both a consumption good that yields direct satisfaction and utility, and an investment good, which yields satisfaction to consumers indirectly through increased productivity, fewer sick days, and higher wages. Investment in health is costly as consumers must trade off time and resources devoted to health, such as exercising at a local gym, against other goals. These factors are used to determine the optimal level of health that an individual will demand. The model makes predictions over the effects of changes in prices of health care and other goods, labour market outcomes such as employment and wages, and technological changes. These predictions and other predictions from models extending Grossman's 1972, the basis of much of the econometric research conducted by health economists.

In Grossman's model, the optimal level of investment in health occurs where the marginal cost of health capital is equal to the marginal benefit. With the passing of time, health depreciates at some rate □. The interest rate faced by the consumer is denoted by r. The marginal cost of health capital can be found by adding these variables: MCHK= r + □. The marginal benefit of health capital is the rate of return from this capital in both market and non-market sectors. In this model, the optimal health stock can be impacted by factors like age, wages and education. As an example, □ increases with age, so it becomes more and more costly to attain the same level of health capital or health stock as one ages. Age also decreases the marginal benefit of health stock. The optimal health stock will therefore decrease as one ages.

Beyond issues of the fundamental, "real" demand for medical care derived from the desire to have good health is the important distinction between the "marginal benefit" of medical care and a separate "effective demand" curve, which summarizes the amount of medical care demanded at particular market prices. Because most medical care is not purchased from providers directly, but is rather obtained at subsidized prices due to insurance, the out-of-pocket prices faced by consumers are typically much lower than the market price.

The consumer sets MB=MC out of pocket, and so the "effective demand" will have a separate relationship between price and quantity than will the "marginal benefit curve" or real demand relationship. This distinction is often described under the rubric of "ex-post moral hazard" (which is again distinct from ex-ante moral hazard, which is found in any type of market with insurance).

ECONOMIC EVALUATION IN THE UNITED KINGDOM

A large focus of health economics, is the microeconomic evaluation of the value of individual treatments. In the UK, the National Institute for Health and Clinical Excellence (NICE) appraises certain new and existing pharmaceuticals and devices using economic evaluation. Economic evaluation is the comparison of two or more alternative courses of action in terms of both their costs and consequences.

Economists usually distinguish several types of economic evaluation, differing in how consequences are measured:

- Cost-minimization analysis
- Cost benefit analysis
- Cost-effectiveness analysis
- Cost-utility analysis

In cost minimization analysis (CMA), the effectiveness of the comparators in question must be proven to be equivalent. The 'cost-effective' comparator is simply the one which costs less (as it achieves the same outcome). In cost-benefit analysis (CBA), costs and benefits are both valued in cash terms. Cost effectiveness analysis (CEA) measures outcomes in 'natural units', such as mmHg, symptom free days, life years gained.

Finally cost-utility analysis (CUA) measures outcomes in a composite metric of both length and quality of life, the Quality-adjusted life year (QALY). (Note there is some international variation in the precise definitions of each type of analysis).

A final approach which is sometimes classed an economic evaluation is a cost of illness study. This is not a true economic evaluation as it does not compare the costs and outcomes of alternative courses of action. Instead, it attempts to measure all the costs associated with a particular disease or condition. These will include direct costs (where money actually changes hands, e.g. health service use, patient co-payments and out of pocket expenses), indirect costs (the value of lost productivity from time off work due to illness), and intangible costs (the 'disvalue' to an individual of pain and suffering).

MARKET EQUILIBRIUM

HEALTH CARE MARKETS

The five health markets typically analysed are:

1. Health care financing market
2. Physician and nurses services market
3. Institutional services market
4. Input factors market
5. Professional education market

Although assumptions of textbook models of economic markets apply reasonably well to health care markets, there are important deviations. Many states have created risk pools in which relatively healthy enrollees subsidise the care of the rest. Insurers must cope with adverse selection which occurs when they are unable to fully predict the medical expenses of enrollees; adverse selection can destroy the risk pool. Features of insurance market risk pools, such as group purchases, preferential selection ("cherry-picking"), and preexisting condition exclusions are meant to cope with adverse selection.

Insured patients are naturally less concerned about health care costs than they would if they paid the full price of care. The resulting moral hazard drives up costs, as shown by the famous RAND Health Insurance Experiment. Insurers use several techniques to limit the costs of moral hazard, including imposing copayments on patients and limiting physician incentives to provide costly care. Insurers often compete by their choice of service offerings, cost sharing requirements, and limitations on physicians.

Consumers in health care markets often suffer from a lack of adequate information about what services they need to buy and which providers offer the best value proposition. Health economists have documented a problem with supplier induced demand, whereby providers base treatment recommendations on economic, rather than medical criteria. Researchers have also documented substantial "practice variations", whereby the treatment aols on service availability to rein in inducement and practice variations.

The U.S. health care market has relied extensively on competition to control costs and improve quality. Critics question whether problems with adverse selection, moral hazard, information asymmetries, demand inducement, and practice variations can be addressed by private markets. Competition has fostered reductions in prices, but consolidation by providers and, to a lesser extent, insurers, has tempered this effect.

Though the market for health care in the U.S. is primarily coordinated by competition, there is an abundance of regulations that inhibit market efficiency. A classic example is medical licenses. Some economists argue that requiring doctors to have a medical license constrains inputs, inhibits innovation, and increases cost to consumers while largely only benefiting the doctors themselves.

COMPETITIVE EQUILIBRIUM IN THE FIVE HEALTH MARKETS

While the nature of health care as a private good is preserved in the last three markets, market failures occur in the financing and delivery markets due to two reasons:

1. Perfect information about price products is not a viable assumption
2. Various barriers of entry exist in the financing markets (i.e. monopoly formations in the insurance industry)

IDEOLOGICAL BIAS IN THE DEBATE ABOUT THE FINANCING AND DELIVERY HEALTH MARKETS

The health care debate in public policy is often informed by ideology and not sound economic theory. Often, politicians subscribe to a moral order system or belief about the role of governments in public life that guides biases towards provision of health care as well. The ideological spectrum spans: individual savings accounts and catastrophic coverage, tax credit or voucher programmes combined with group purchasing arrangements, and expansions of public- sector health insurance. These approaches are advocated by health care conservatives, moderates and liberals, respectively.

OTHER ISSUES

MEDICAL ECONOMICS

Often used synonymously with Health Economics, Medical economics, according to Culyer, is the branch of economics concerned with the application of economic theory to phenomena and problems associated typically with the second and third health market. Typically, however, it pertains to cost-benefit analysis of pharmaceutical products and cost- effectiveness of various medical treatments. Medical economics often uses math-ematical models to synthesise data from biostatistics and epidemiology for support of medical decision making, both for individuals and for wider health policy.

BEHAVIOURAL ECONOMICS

Peter Orszag has suggested that behavioural economics is an important factor for improving the health care system, but that relatively little progress has been made when compared to retirement policy.

MENTAL HEALTH ECONOMICS

Mental health economics incorporates a vast array of subject matters, ranging from pharmacoeconomics to labour and welfare economics. Mental health can be directly related to economics by the potential of affected individuals to contribute as human capital. In 2009 Currie and Stabile published "Mental Health in Childhood and Human Capital" in which they assessed how common childhood mental health problems may alter the human capital accumulation of affected children.

Externalities may include the influence that affected individuals have on surrounding human capital, such as at the workplace or in the home. In turn, the economy also affects the individual, particularly in light of globalization. For example, studies in India, where there is an increasingly high occurrence of western outsourcing, have demonstrated a growing hybrid identity in young professionals who face very different sociocultural expectations at the workplace and in at home.

Mental health economics presents a unique set of challenges to researchers. In health economics, the health status of an individual may be given a value such as HYE (Health Year Equivalents); however, in mental health economics, valuations may not be the same for affected individuals.

For instance a suicidal individual may place higher utility on death than life. Additionally, individuals with cognitive disabilities may not be able to communicate preferences.

These factors represent challenges in terms of placing value on the mental health status of an individual, especially in relation to the individual's potential as human capital. Further, employment statistics are often used in mental health economic studies as a means of evaluating individual productivity; however, these statistics do not capture "presenteeism", when an individual is at work with a lowered productivity level, quantify the loss of non-paid working time, or capture externalities such as having an affected family member. Also, considering the variation in global wage rates or in societal values, statistics used may be contextually, geo-graphically confined, and study results may not be inter-nationally applicable.

Though studies have demonstrated mental health care to reduce overall health care costs, demonstrate efficacy, and reduce employee absenteeism while improving employee functioning, the availability of comprehensive mental health services is in decline.

Petrasek and Rapin cite the three main reasons for this decline as:

1. Stigma and privacy concerns,
2. The difficulty of quantifying medical savings and
3. Physician incentive to medicate without specialist referral.

Evers have suggested that improvements could be made by promoting more active dissemination of mental health economic analysis, building partnerships through policy-makers and researchers, and employing greater use of knowledge brokers.

HEALTH CARE IN INDIA

Health care in India is the responsibility of constituent states and territories of India. The Constitution charges every state with "raising of the level of nutrition and the standard of living of its people and the improvement of public health as among its primary duties". The National Health Policy was endorsed by the Parliament of India in 1983 and updated in 2002.

The art of Health Care in India can be traced back nearly 3500 years. From the early days of Indian history the Aryurvedic tradition of medicine has been practiced. During the rule of Emperor Ashoka Maurya (third century B.C.E.), schools of learning in the healing arts were created. Many valuable herbs and medicinal combinations were created. Even today many of these continue to be used. During his rein there is evidence that Emperor Ashoka was the first leader in world history to attempt to give health care to all of his citizens, thus it was the India of antiquity which was the first state to give it's citizens national health care.

In recent times India has eradicated mass famines, half of children in India are underweight, one of the highest rates in the world and nearly the same rate of Sub-Saharan Africa. Water supply and sanitation in India continue to be a challenge, only one of three Indians has access to improved sanitation facilities such as toilet. India's HIV/AIDS epidemic is a growing threat. Cholera epidemics are not unknown. The maternal mortality in India is the second highest in the world.

Providing health care and disease prevention to India's growing population of more than a billion people becomes challenging in the face of increased competition for resources. 2.47 million people in India are estimated to be HIV positive. India is one of the four countries worldwide where polio has not as yet been successfully eradicated and one third of the world's tuberculosis cases are in India. Three out of four children who died from measles in 2008 were in India. According to the World Health Organization 900,000 Indians die each year from drinking contaminated water and breathing in polluted air. As India grapples with these basic issues, new challenges are emerging for example there is a rise in chronic adult diseases such as cardiovascular illnesses and diabetes as a consequence of changing lifestyles.

There are vast disparities in people's health even among the different states across the country largely attributed to the resource allocation by the state governments where some states have been more successful than others. Critics say better efforts are needed by the local governments to ensure that the health services provided are actually reaching the poor in worst-affected areas.

However, at the same time, India's health care system also includes entities which are world class. India is a magnet for medical tourists, who are able to get medical treatments and surgeries at a fraction of the cost of these procedures in developed countries. The Apollo set of hospitals, for example, thrives on this business. Each hospital, however, must also set aside a number of beds for the poor. However, as the BBC reported, access to these services by the poor is plagued with corruption. While many foreign medical experts criticize medical tourism, many private hospitals are able to demonstrate that their level of care is comparable, if not better, than that received in developed countries.

MEDICAL PROFESSIONALS

In a 2005 World Bank study, World Bank reported that "a detailed survey of the knowledge of medical practitioners for treating five common conditions in Delhi found that the average doctor in a public primary health centre has around a 50-50 chance of recommending a harmful treatment". Random visits by government inspectors showed that 40% of public sector medical workers were not found at the workplace.

NEUROSURGERY

Modern neurosurgery in India begins in 1949, with the return of Jacob Chandy to the Christian Medical College, Vellore. Stereotactic surgery for pain, epilepsy, behaviour disorders and involuntary movements is being practised at several centres especially at Madras. As of 1983, there were about 180 neurosurgeons in India, or one for 3.6 million people.

DISEASES

Ongoing government of India education about HIV has led to decreases in the spread of HIV in recent years. The number of people living with AIDS in India is estimated to be between 2 and 3 million. However in terms of the total population this is a small number. The country has had a sharp decrease in the estimated number of HIV infections; 2005 reports had claimed that there were 5.2 million to 5.7 million people afflicted with the virus.

MALNUTRITION

Half of children in India are underweight, one of the highest rates in the world and nearly same as Sub-Saharan Africa. India contributes to about 5.6 million child deaths every year, more than half the world's total.

WOMEN

Most Indian women are malnourished. The average female life expectancy today in India is low compared to many countries, but it has shown gradual improvement over the years. In many families, especially rural ones, the girls and women face nutritional discrimination within the family, and are anemic and malnourished.

The maternal mortality in India is the second highest in the world. Only 42% of births in the country are supervised by health professionals. Most women deliver with help from women in the family who often lack the skills and resources to save the mother's life if it is in danger. According to UNDP Human Development Report (1997), 88% of pregnant women (age 15-49) were found to be suffering from anemia.

WATER AND SANITATION

Water supply and sanitation in India continue to be abysmal, despite longstanding efforts by the various levels of government and communities at improving coverage. The situation is particularly inadequate for sanitation, since only one of three Indians has access to improved sanitation facilities (including improved latrines).

While the share of those with access to an improved water source is much higher than for sanitation (86%), the quality of service is poor and most users that are counted as having access receive water of dubious quality and only on an intermittent basis. As of 2003, it was estimated that only 30% of India's wastewater was being treated, with the remainder flowing into rivers or groundwater.

The lack of toilet facilities in many areas also presents a major health risk; open defecation is widespread even in urban areas of India, and it was estimated in 2002 by the World Health Organisation that around 700,000

Indians die each year from diarrhoea. No city in India has full-day water supply. Most cities supply water only a few hours a day. In towns and rural areas the situation is even worse.

HEALTH CARE INFRASTRUCTURE

The Indian health care industry is seen to be growing at a rapid pace and is expected to become a Us." billion industry by 2022. The Indian health care market was estimated at US$35 billion in 2007 and is expected to reach over US$70 billion by 2012 and Us." billion by 2017.

According to the Investment Commission of India the health care sector has experienced phenomenal growth of 12 percent per annum in the last 4 years. Rising income levels and a growing elderly population are all factors that are driving this growth. In addition, changing demographics, disease profiles and the shift from chronic to lifestyle diseases in the country has led to increased spending on health care delivery.

Even so, the vast majority of the country suffers from a poor standard of health care infrastructure which has not kept up with the growing economy. Despite having centres of excellence in health care delivery, these facilities are limited and are inadequate in meeting the current health care demands. Most public health facilities lack efficiency, are understaffed and have poorly maintained or outdated medical equipment.

Approximately one million people, mostly women and children, die in India each year due to inadequate health care. 700 million people have no access to specialist care and 80% of specialists live in urban areas. In addition to poor infrastructure India faces a shortage of trained medical personal especially in rural areas where access to care is altogether limited.

In order to meet manpower shortages and reach world standards India would require investments of up to $20 billion over the next 5 years. Forty percent of the primary health centres in India are understaffed. According to WHO statistics there are over 250 medical colleges in the modern system of medicine and over 400 in the Indian system of medicine and homeopathy (ISM&H).

India produces over 250,000 doctors annually in the modern system of medicine and a similar number of ISM&H practitioners, nurses and para professionals. Better policy regulations and the establishment of public private partnerships are possible solutions to the problem of manpower shortage. India faces a huge need gap in terms of availability of number of hospital beds per 1000 population. With a world average of 3.96 hospital beds per 1000 population India stands just a little over 0.7 hospital beds per 1000 population.

Moreover, India faces a shortage of doctors, nurses and paramedics that are needed to propel the growing health care industry. India is now looking at establishing academic medical centres (AMCs) for the delivery of higher quality care with leading examples of The Manipal Group & All India Institute of Medical Sciences (AIIMS) already in place.

As incomes rise and the number of available financing options in terms of health insurance policies increase, consumers become more and more engaged in making informed decisions about their health and are well aware of the costs associated with those decisions. In order to remain competitive, health care providers are now not only looking at improving operational efficiency but are also looking at ways of enhancing patient experience overall.

CENTRAL GOVERNMENT ROLE

Critics say that the national policy lacks specific measures to achieve broad stated goals. Particular problems include the failure to integrate health services with wider economic and social development, the lack of nutritional support and sanitation, and the poor participatory involvement at the local level. Central government efforts at influencing public health have focused on the five-year plans, on coordinated planning with the states, and on sponsoring major health programmes. Government expenditures are jointly shared by the central and state governments.

Goals and strategies are set through central-state government consultations of the Central Council of Health and Family Welfare. Central government efforts are administered by the Ministry of Health and Family Welfare, which provides both administrative and technical services and manages medical education. States provide public services and health education.

The 1983 National Health Policy is committed to providing health services to all by 2000. In 1983 health care expenditures varied greatly among the states and union territories, from ₹ 13 per capita in Bihar to ₹ 60 per capita in Himachal Pradesh, and Indian per capita expenditure was low when compared with other Asian countries outside of South Asia. Although government health care spending progressively grew throughout the 1980s, such spending as a percentage of the gross national product (GNP) remained fairly constant. In the meantime, health care spending as a share of total government spending decreased. During the same period, private-sector spending on health care was about 1.5 times as much as government spending.

EXPENDITURE

In the mid-1990s, health spending amounted to 6% of GDP, one of the highest levels among developing nations. The established per capita spending is around ₹ 320 per year with the major input from private households (75%).

State governments contribute 15.2%, the central government 5.2%, third- party insurance and employers 3.3%, and municipal government and foreign donors about 1.3, according to a 1995 World Bank study. Of these proportions, 58.7% goes towards primary health care (curative, preventive, and promotive) and 38.8% is spent on secondary and tertiary inpatient care. The rest goes for non-service costs.

The fifth and sixth five-year plans (FY 1974-78 and FY 1980-84, respectively) included programmes to assist delivery of preventive medicine and improve the health status of the rural population. Supplemental nutrition programmes and increasing the supply of safe drinking water were high priorities. The sixth plan aimed at training more community health workers and increasing efforts to control communicable diseases. There were also efforts to improve regional imbalances in the distribution of health care resources.

The Seventh Five-Year Plan (FY 1985-89) budgeted ₹ 33.9 billion for health, an amount roughly double the outlay of the sixth plan. Health spending as a portion of total plan outlays, however, had declined over the years since the first plan in 1951, from a high of 3.3% of the total plan spending in FY 1951-55 to 1.9% of the total for the seventh plan. Mid-way through the Eighth Five- Year Plan (FY 1992-96), however, health and family welfare was budgeted at ₹ 20 billion, or 4.3% of the total plan spending for FY 1994, with an additional ₹ 3.6 billion in the non-plan budget.

PRIMARY SERVICES

Health care facilities and personnel increased substantially between the early 1950s and early 1980s, but because of fast population growth, the number of licensed medical practitioners per 10,000 individuals had fallen by the late 1980s to three per 10,000 from the 1981 level of four per 10,000. In 1991 there were approximately ten hospital beds per 10,000 individuals. However for comparison, the in China for comparison there are 1.4 doctors per 1000 people.

Primary health centres are the cornerstone of the rural health care system. By 1991, India had about 22,400 primary health centres, 11,200 hospitals, and 27,400 clinics. These facilities are part of a tiered health care system that funnels more difficult cases into urban hospitals while attempting to provide routine medical care to the vast majority in the countryside.

Primary health centres and subcenters rely on trained paramedics to meet most of their needs. The main problems affecting the success of primary health centres are the predominance of clinical and curative concerns over the intended emphasis on preventive work and the reluctance of staff to work in rural areas. In addition, the integration of health services with family planning programmes often causes the local population to perceive the primary health centres as hostile to their traditional preference for large families. Therefore, primary health centres often play an adversarial role in local efforts to implement national health policies.

According to data provided in 1989 by the Ministry of Health and Family Welfare, the total number of civilian hospitals for all states and union territories combined was 10,157. In 1991 there was a total of 811,000 hospital and health care facilities beds. The geographical distribution of hospitals varied according to local socio-economic conditions. In India's most populous state, Uttar Pradesh, with a 1991 population of more than 139 million, there were 735 hospitals as of 1990. In Kerala, with a 1991 population of 29 million occupying an area only one-seventh the size of Uttar Pradesh, there were 2,053 hospitals.

Although central government has set a goal of health care for all by 2000, hospitals are distributed unevenly. Private studies of India's total number of hospitals in the early 1990s were more conservative than official Indian data, estimating that in 1992 there were 7,300 hospitals.

Of this total, nearly 4,000 were owned and managed by central, state, or local governments. Another 2,000, owned and managed by charitable trusts, received partial support from the government, and the remaining 1,300 hospitals, many of which were relatively small facilities, were owned and managed by the private sector. The use of state-of-the-art medical equipment, often imported from Western countries, was primarily limited to urban centres in the early 1990s.

A network of regional cancer diagnostic and treatment facilities was being established in the early 1990s in major hospitals that were part of government medical colleges. By 1992 twenty-two such centres were in operation. Most of the 1,300 private hospitals lacked sophisticated medical facilities, although in 1992 approximately 12% possessed state-of-the-art equipment for diagnosis and treatment of all major diseases, including cancer. The fast pace of development of the private medical sector and the burgeoning middle class in the 1990s have led to the emergence of the new concept in India of establishing hospitals and health care facilities on a for-profit basis.

By the late 1980s, there were approximately 128 medical colleges - roughly three times more than in 1950. These medical colleges in 1987 accepted a combined annual class of 14,166 students. Data for 1987 show that there were 320,000 registered medical practitioners and 219,300 registered nurses. Various studies have shown that in both urban and rural areas people preferred to pay and seek the more sophisticated services provided by private physicians rather than use free treatment at public health centres. Indigenous or traditional medical practitioners continue to practice throughout the country. The two main forms of traditional medicine practised are the ayurvedic system, which deals with mental and spiritual as well as physical well-being, and the unani (or Galenic) herbal medical practice. A vaidya is a practitioner of the ayurvedic tradition, and a hakim is a practitioner of the unani or Greek tradition.

These professions are frequently hereditary. A variety of institutions offer training in indigenous medical practice. Only in the late 1970s did official health policy refer to any form of integration between European-trained medical personnel and indigenous medical practitioners. In the early 1990s, there were ninety-eight ayurvedic colleges and seventeen unani colleges operating in both the governmental and non-governmental sectors.

HEALTH INSURANCE

The majority of the Indian population is unable to access high quality health care provided by private players as a result of high costs. Many are now looking towards insurance companies for providing alternative financing options so that they too may seek better quality health care.

The opportunity remains huge for insurance providers entering into the Indian health care market since75% of expenditure on health care in India is still being met by 'out-of-pocket' consumers. Even though only 10% of the Indian population today has health insurance coverage, this industry is expected to face tremendous growth over the next few years as a result of several private players that have entered into the market.

Health insurance coverage among urban, middle- and upper-class Indians, however, is significantly higher and stands at approximately 50%. The Insurance Regulatory and Development Authority (IRDA) is the governing body responsible for promoting insurance business and introducing insurance regulations in India.

The share of public sector companies in health insurance premiums was 76% and that of private sector companies was 24% for the period 2005-06. Health insurance premiums collected over 2005-06 registered a growth of 35% over the previous year. In 2001 the IRDA introduced provisions for Third Party Administrators (TPAs) to support the administration and management of health insurance products offered by insurance companies. TPAs are facilitators in the coordination process between the health insurance provider and the hospital. Currently there are 27 TPAs registered under the IRDA.

Health insurance has a way of increasing accessibility to quality health care delivery especially for private health care providers for whom high cost remains a barrier. In order to encourage foreign health insurers to enter the Indian market the government has recently proposed to raise the foreign direct investment (FDI) limit in insurance from 26% to 49%. Increasing health insurance penetration and ensuring affordable premium rates are necessary to drive the health insurance market in India.

MEDICAL TOURISM

India is becoming a location for medical tourists seeking health care at lower costs than in other countries.

RATE OF GROWTH

India has approximately 600,000 allopathic doctors registered to practice medicine. This number however, is higher than the actual number practicing because it includes doctors who have emigrated to other countries as well as doctors who have died. India licenses 18,000 new doctors a year.

FUNDING HEALTH CARE SERVICES

The Wanless Report, published in 2002, highlighted that in order to secure an improvement in the quality of the services provided in the UK, expenditure on health care services would have to increase towards 12% of gross domestic product (GDP) - an increase from the current £68 billion to well over £150 billion (2002/03 prices) on the best estimates and over £180 billion when less favourable estimates are used.

However, the resources available for health services (public or private) are finite and the health care dilemma forces governments and decision-makers to make choices, which at times are extremely difficult. The ever-increasing demand for health care services against a background of limited resources - emphasised by current shortages among doctors - that is likely to be exacerbated during the foreseeable future as fewer people apply for places in medical schools has been addressed by a number of broad policy options, with varying degrees of success. These are briefly outlined below.

INCREASE EFFICIENCY

This option covers a whole variety of themes ranging from reducing the costs of catering or domestic services (through competitive tendering) to reducing the unit costs of treating patients through, for example, a move from inpatient surgery to day case surgery. The overall aim is the same, to get the health care services to deliver more care for the same amount of money. Broadly speaking, the recent reforms to the NHS in the UK have been primarily concerned with promoting greater efficiency in service delivery. However, the drive for greater efficiency may result in equity in health having to be compromised.

LIMIT SERVICE RANGE

The term prioritisation or its negative version, rationalisation, have become part of everyday usage within health care systems in recent years. As a process, it is an 'elaborate and intricate issue' and also highly emotive. For example, the funding of the so-called 'lifestyle drug' Viagra became one of the major elements in debates surrounding the rationing of health care interventions.

The government argued that the mechanisms of funding this type of intervention might even threaten the financial sustainability of current health systems, with the Secretary of State for Health making the case that, with regard to clinical need, impotence could not be regarded as a priority for any additional NHS expenditure compared with cancer, heart disease and mental health since, while it may result in psychological distress, it was not life- threatening or causing physical pain.

Another example of the issues revolving around establishing priorities was found in the case of child B, a ten-year-old girl suffering from acute myeloid leukaemia. After a bone marrow transplant, the disease appeared to have been cured but the leukaemia returned and clinicians told the girl's father that she had only a few weeks to live. He contacted a private practitioner who was willing to treat child B with a new treatment that would cost £75 000.

The HA refused to fund the treatment or provide a second bone marrow transplant since expert opinion was that the chances of success were extremely slim. A high-profile legal battle ensued and eventually the Court of Appeal found in favour of the HA. An anonymous benefactor provided the funds for the treatment and the girl survived for another year before a further relapse led to her death. Although this particular example achieved national media attention, priority-setting decisions involving ethical and other costeffective considerations are at the heart of policies and local decision-making on an everyday basis.

The establishment of NICE sought to address the problems associated with 'postcode prescribing', where services and treatments were available in one area but not in a neighbouring location. Before NICE the process of limiting the range of services made available had been ad hoc and not without considerable controversy, as evidenced in the two examples above, but the extent to which NICE has succeeded has yet to be proved.

ADDITIONAL FUNDING

The option favoured by most NHS staff and, according to opinion polls, by a large proportion of the general public would be to increase the level of funds going into the existing NHS. This could be done in a number of ways, such as levying charges, increasing taxation proceeds or shifting resources from other parts of the public sector.

What is not evident, however, is the extent to which additional resources will translate into additional health benefits, and to whom they would accrue. Additional resources may prove to be very welcome but if they are channelled into inappropriate areas, the result may be greater inefficiency and wider inequalities. The contrasting situations in terms of expenditure and indicators of health status from the USA and Japan, while the comparison between the NHS and Kaiser Permanente also challenge such a view. The question is whether additional resources to improve job prospects and reduce poverty, for example, would result in greater health care benefits than would be gained from additional expenditure on health care facilities and treatments.

ALTERNATIVE FINANCING STRUCTURE

A fourth alternative would be to completely restructure the method of organising and funding health services. In the UK, this could involve the deployment of some form of health insurance system. For example, 500 hospital consultants issued a call for the radical reform of the NHS to put power into patients' hands, by taking out a full-page advertisement in The Times on 25 February 2004.

The group, entitled Doctors for Reform, stated their commitment to the NHS ideals of equitable and universal health care but believed that this could be better achieved by other methods of financing. Professor Karol Sikora, an oncologist and one of the founder members of the group, said:

The NHS as we know it has had its day. You can fiddle about with it and patch it up, but with an ageing population and high-tech health care, something has to give. Everything else we need today we can get very easily: air travel, holidays, cars. Why can't we get health care that easily? The form of funding is the key. To change it is a radical step. Politicians are very nervous. But we have to do it if we want a system that is focused on the patient and open to innovative ideas. However, there is no guarantee that changes in the financing structures willgenerate improvement in performance. While there is some evidence of excess demand for health care services and insufficient supply of health care resources in the UK compared to other countries - for example, it was shown that UK had 50% of the number of beds per 1000 population compared to France in 200044 - many of the problems that face the NHS in the UK and health systems in other countries are not primarily a function of their funding arrangements.

They are in fact multifactorial, resulting from factors such as external cost pressures on pharmaceuticals and other medical equipment and devices, growing demands from an expanding and increasingly articulate and informed population, and pressures on the supply of human resources resulting from demographic changes and legislation relating to working conditions.

The World Health Organization (WHO) produced a report in 2000 that sought to establish criteria to assess the performance of health care systems across the world. The five goals against which each health care system was to be judged were maximisation of population health, reducing inequalities in the health of populations, maximising responsiveness, reducing inequalities in responsiveness and financing health care in a fair manner.

However, while the intention was generally sound and there was considerable analysis to support the work, the quality of the underlying database was of dubious quality, with an excessive reliance on estimates. What is evident is that it is extremely difficult to identify which health systems are the most efficient46,47 and which secure the greatest 'benefit per buck' for its residents.

REDUCE DEMAND FOR HEALTH SERVICES

A key policy plank of most governments would be to try and reduce the demand for health services by preventing people from getting ill in the first place. It has been estimated that preventable illness constitutes approximately 70% of the burden of illness and the associated costs and therefore the incentives to utilise health promotion and preventive measures for such a purpose are obviously attractive.

However, there are two basic issues at stake: firstly, is there evidence that prevention and health promotion reduce health care costs; and secondly, whether any health care programme or intervention should be assessed in relation to its impact on financial budgets? In response to the first it is surely the prime objective of any health care intervention or programme to improve the health of the particular patients or community, which as a result may secure reductions in costs to the health service and patients and communities. The same principle should apply to any consideration of prevention and health promotion, and the more appropriate question is whether additional resources spent on prevention or health promotion would generate greater health benefits than if those resources had been used elsewhere?

The second issue has grown in importance recently as purchasers have to operate within constrained budgets. The publication of guidance and guidelines, even when based on quality evidence, can have a profound impact on available resources. For example, it was argued that implementation of the guidance on statins in patients at high risk of coronary heart disease could potentially cost a single HA in the UK roughly 20% of its annual drug budget.

While health economic evaluation can be utilised in decisions relating to the prioritisation of services, it is not sufficient to predict whether they are affordable within available budgets. It is becoming usual for budget impact assessment to be included alongside economic evaluations when evidence is submitted to agencies deciding on formulary inclusion or reimbursement.

More attention is devoted to this process in the plethora of different forms of health care systems around the world, with their different forms of financing and organising the delivery of health care services, seems to imply that there is no single, unique or right way of doing things. It could also mean that different systems have evolved to suit different societies with different cultures, ideas and notions of medicine, the citizen's right to care and so on. What is evident, however, is that systems are continually changing and evolving. So how much should be spent on health and health care? Who should decide?

EXPENDITURE ON HEALTH CARE SERVICES

There is considerable variation between countries in the levels of health care expenditure. However, it does not necessarily mean that countries at the top of the chart, with a greater share of their GDP allocated to health, have the best returns from such expenditure and those at the bottom have the worst, as evidenced by the comparison made between the situations in Japan and the USA. There is a distinction made between public sector and private sector health care expenditure, but this, in many senses, is an oversimplification. For example, within the UK, certain medication is available over the counter at the local pharmacist, but only some people are entitled to 'free' treatments as prescribed by their GP. The same distinctions apply to aspects of dental care, ophthalmic services, etc., where some sections of the population receive the services without having to pay directly, while others have to pay the full amount. Distinctions and differences also apply in other countries, with some people entitled to full reimbursement on any costs incurred in treatments, while others are only entitled to a percentage of the full amount.

DIFFERENT APPROACHES TO FINANCING

There are in essence four basic alternative methods of financing care services:

1. Direct payment by users
2. Private health insurance
3. Social or state insurance
4. Direct tax

All health care systems are essentially pluralistic with respect to financing (and delivery), with tendencies towards one method rather than another. For example, in the USA the health care economy is dominated by private health insurance but with a significant proportion of government-funded care, while in Switzerland, 25% of total health expenditure comes from social insurance, 33% from direct payments and 40% from general taxes. Consideration was given to the concept of health as distinguished from health care, and the idea propounded that by spending more on factors external to the health care system less would be required by the health care system. Obviously this question is addressed to the notion of state funding rather than any individual decision to purchase more health and social care. Four practical approaches have been suggested to the problem of determining the level of state funding of health and social care.

They are:

1. Incremental funding
2. Incremental funding linked to affordability
3. International comparisons
4. Democratic decision

INCREMENTAL FUNDING

This approach involves looking at current levels of expenditure and then making some changes at the margin to produce a new budget for the next year. However, with this approach no account is taken of the allocation of funds within the system; demographic changes are not considered; medical advances and technological changes are ignored; health policy developments are not taken into consideration; and any fundamental underfunding of the system is not dealt with.

INCREMENTAL FUNDING LINKED TO AFFORDABILITY

Such an approach ties increases in health care expenditure to increases in the wealth of the nation - GDP. Hence, one would expect public expenditure on health and social care to be a constant percentage of GDP. However, there are two major problems with this approach. Firstly, what happens when GDP is falling or only rising marginally? There is evidence to suggest that demand for health care resources increases during recessionary periods, which suggests that the relationship between health expenditure and GDP is inverse. Should this be reflected in the way health expenditure levels are tied to GDP or should there be a minimum baseline growth in health expenditure, which negates the rationale for a GDP linkage?

The second criticism relates to the political implications for governments in seeking to tie health care expenditure to GDP growth. It is highly unlikely that any government would willingly surrender their control of a proportion of public spending to a formula that dictated spending levels. Furthermore, there may well be pressure to encourage private health expenditure and reduce the burden on the public purse, as well as from private sector providers themselves, to increase 'market share', to maintain parity with GDP.

The distributive effects of such a policy would in all probability exacerbate inequalities in health care as private health care would not be attainable for the low paid, high risk and uninsurable.

INTERNATIONAL COMPARISONS

This is an oft-quoted statistic but one which is very unreliable as an indicator. Not only is it difficult to collect comparable data but interpreting the data and drawing conclusions from such data are highly susceptible to criticisms (e.g. cultural factors, differences in definitions, differences in demographic and epidemiological patterns).

Other issues arise due to the nature of comparisons made. For example, currency fluctuations can result in major changes in comparisons without any actual change in expenditure. An alternative approach has been the use of purchasing power parities, which relate to the cost of health care to the economy as a whole, having made allowance for differences in the level of general prices between countries.

However, differences in the price of health care products and services are not necessarily accounted for, and so another approach has been to employ health care- specific purchasing power parities. The reliability of these data and the complexities and differences between health care systems means that extreme caution should be taken in using international comparisons in seeking to establish the appropriate level of spending on health care.

DEMOCRATIC DECISION

The issue surrounding levels of health care expenditure is essentially a normative one, based on value judgements. Within democracies the voting system, in theory at least, is the means by which difficult issues involving value judgements can be resolved. However, in reality this is often not the case.

A number of government policies are not necessarily contained within election manifestos and therefore do not appear before the electorate for their consideration and approval. In addition the question of who votes is very important. A number of groups within society are disenfranchised, some of whom are heavy users of resources in health and social care, while others are unable to vote because of disability, infirmity, etc.

Opinion polls are alternative ways of acquiring the views of society but these suffer from methodological problems, and while there are some examples of community-wide surveys and ballots relating to the issue of funding health and social care, there is no evidence to date of them penetrating into political agendas.

The inadequacies of outcome measures also compound the problems in seeking to reach a consensus as to what level of funding is appropriate, and one is left with the inevitable conclusion that if democracy is to have any say in the arguments, it hinges on the amount of imperfection that one is prepared to tolerate in the information available and in the methodologies used to acquire the views of the community. The question as to how much should actually be spent on health care services was addressed at a conference following publication of the Wanless Report. It is worth quoting the conclusion reached by the editors of the publication resulting from the conference:

As already alluded to, it is not possible to reduce a review of future spending to a technical exercise (albeit a very complicated one) (i.e the Wanless review). There are questions of value (particularly in a non-marketed service such as the NHS) which are best addressed not by economists, politicians or Treasury policy wonks, but by society more generally. There are also prior questions about the sort of NHS we want - the 'vision' - and what we are prepared to sacrifice in order to achieve it. No amount of modelling, no matter how sophisticated, will help answer such vital questions - rather, they require consideration by those to whom the NHS is ultimately accountable: the public and patients.

❐

Chapter - 6

Hospitals of Future Generation

INTRODUCTION

Human lives weigh in the balance every day in hospitals. For hospital patients and their families, the hospital experience is often a central point in their life – where their child was born, their beloved died, where they received life-saving treatment, rejuvenating therapy or care to overcome an episode of illness. The hospital is the setting of oft-told tales among friends and family through the generations. It is no wonder that hospitals are often used to depict human drama – and even comedy — for popular consumption across the panorama of entertainment media. In reality, hospitals are the setting where cutting-edge medical advances relieve suffering, and bring healing and even new life for those whom, even a few short years ago, there would be little hope. Featherweight babies, born eight weeks prematurely can now survive and even thrive.

Minimally invasive surgeries allow patients to heal quickly with less risk of complication, and speed their journey home. The evolving science of organ transplantation brings a second shot at life for an increasing number of people whose lives would otherwise be foreshortened. In addition to their impact on human life, hospitals are a major driver of the U.S. economy. The hospital industry is the second largest private-sector employer in the U.S. and contributes nearly $2 trillion of economic activity. In many small communities across the country, the local hospital is the largest employer and most valuable economic asset. Consumer attitude towards hospitals waxes and wanes, seemingly with some dependence on hospital news that makes headlines, such as traumatic medical errors, rampant hospital-acquired infection, and unscrupulous billing practices. There is no doubt that hospitals face greater scrutiny over the issues that can erode public trust. In order to secure the public's trust, hospitals will need to become highly reliable — ensuring patients' safety, providing clinically effective care, and embodying the ethical ideal that has long been the expectation of the public. Hospitals will have to meet the high expectations of the public and all stakeholders in an increasingly challenging environment. There are many issues with which hospitals must now contend.

These include escalating health care costs that are no longer publicly – or politically – tenable, changing trends in reimbursement for services, demands for transparency of cost and quality data, and workforce shortages. At the same time, the conditions and care needs of hospitalized patients are more complex. The rise in patients with chronic illness, older age adults, and medical interventions and therapies, are already influencing hospitals today and that influence will deepen well into the future. The importance of hospital-based care will not diminish in the future. However, changes in the social and economic environments in which hospitals operate, as well as medical and technological progress require hospitals to be equally transformative as the future unfolds. There has been a hospital building boom underway – fueled by increasing demand for health care services and increasingly obsolete hospital plants.

Though economic conditions are expected to slow its pace, the continuing investment in hospital construction offers the opportunity to remake the hospital — its design, culture and practices – to better meet the needs of patients and families and the aspirations of those that provide their care. But, unless there are principles to guide the development of the hospital of the future, hospitals may simply freeze into place the status quo of today. In order to identify these principles, The Joint Commission appointed an expert Roundtable panel comprising hospital administrative and clinical leaders, as well as experts in technology, health care economics, hospital design and patient safety. The Roundtable was charged to evaluate the current health care environment and identify the elements of the future hospital that will position it to play an appropriate role or roles in meeting the needs of patients and publics. Among specific issues that were addressed by the Roundtable were socio-economic trends, technology, the physical environment of care, patient-centered care values, ongoing staffing challenges, and the global confluence of these issues and their impact on the hospital of the future.

ECONOMIC IMPLICATIONS FOR THE HOSPITAL OF THE FUTURE

THE HIGH COST OF DOING BUSINESS

In 2007, the national expenditure on health care was over $2.2 trillion, or $7,500 per U.S. resident. Health care spending accounts for 16.2 percent of Gross Domestic Product (GDP). More than onethird of national health spending is for hospital care, compared to approximately 20 percent for physician services and 10 percent for pharmaceuticals. While health care costs are rising globally, in no country are costs rising at the high rate of those of the U.S. Overall, U.S. per capita health care spending is more than 50 percent higher than any other country. Among the most significant reasons for this contrast are higher income and higher medical prices in the U.S. Indeed, the U.S. pays much higher prices for pharmaceuticals, hospital stays and physician visits.

For its level of investment, the U.S. does not receive a more favourable rate of return as far as higher quality care, patient satisfaction or population health status compared to other industrialized nations. Higher health care costs that are borne by health care purchasers, payers, and consumers are becoming untenable. As a result, health care purchasers are focusing on health benefit cost containment strategies, mainly by shifting more of the cost burden to employees. Job-based health insurance premiums rose 10-times faster than incomes from 2001 to 2005, according to a report from the Robert Wood Johnson Foundation. The amount employees paid for family coverage rose 30 percent, while their incomes rose by three percent. Fewer private- sector businesses offer coverage (-30,000) and as a result, 4.1 million fewer employees are working in private-sector jobs that offer health insurance. Overall, 2.4 million fewer people have private health insurance, a drop of six percent. Year to year more people are uninsured. Today, that figure stands at approximately 47 million people. Meanwhile, public health insurance programmes are experiencing the squeeze of the current economic scenario. High health care costs, a poorly performing U.S. economy, diminished tax revenue, a booming Medicare-eligible generation, as well as growing ranks of uninsured are factors in the expected insolvency of the Medicare programme by 2019.

MORE RED THAN ROSY

While many hospitals are today enjoying relative prosperity – in one survey, hospital systems reported an increase in patient revenues of nearly 8.5 percent in 2007 from the previous year — the conditions upon which these gains are made are expected to dramatically change in the coming years. And, while some hospitals experience healthy profit margins, an uncomfortable number of hospitals continue to be unprofitable. There is a growing gap between have and have-not hospitals that may very well widen as the future unfolds. Hospitals are not invulnerable to current economic conditions. While health care has long been thought to be "recession-proof" because of an endless supply of sick patients and reliance on government payment, health care organizations are as vulnerable to the tightened credit market as any industry. According to a report in Modern Health care, even before the economy started to falter this year, hospital and health system bond rating downgrades were on the upswing, while upgrades were on the downswing. In fact, about 50 percent of shortterm, acute-care hospitals are either insolvent or near insolvency, according to a recent report from Alvarez & Marshal Health care Industry Group. Financial issues are mainly arising from the instability of funding sources, including government subsidies and charitable contributions. Moreover, hospital capital expenses are underfunded by up to $20 billion. By and large, many hospitals are able to achieve a positive bottom-line through cost-shifting – subsidizing services that do not cover costs with more favourable remunerative services.

For treating Medicare patients, hospitals receive $.91 of every dollar expended; for Medicaid patients they receive $.86 per dollar. Uncompensated care accounts for approximately six percent of hospital costs on average – in 2006 that amounted to $30 billion. Yet, from private payers, hospitals receive $1.22 for every dollar spent. Hospitals depend on having robust numbers of privately insured patients in order to be able to treat the under- and uninsured and still remain in the black. This scenario will be increasingly difficult to sustain. With the demographic trend pointing to a growing elderly population, hospitals can expect to have more Medicare patients. Absent any major health reform, with the continuing decline in employer-sponsored insurance and unabated growth in the numbers of uninsured, hospitals can expect more Medicaid patients and uncompensated care. In essence, there will be more competition for the fewer patients to whom costs may be shifted. There is another wrinkle in the cross-subsidy fabric. In order to address escalating health care costs, stakeholders are demanding transparency of the costs and quality of care.

For its part, the federal government has been taking steps to encourage price and quality transparency as one way to spur competition and encourage value-based health care purchasing decisions. An August 2006 Executive Order requires federal agencies that administer or sponsor health programmes to make information available to consumers on the quality and costs of services provided by doctors and hospitals. The Executive Order also requires agencies and their contractors to promote the use of interoperable health care information technology products so that data can easily be shared. The Order further requires federal agencies to offer health insurance programmes that reward consumers who choose health care providers based on value and quality. Based on the Executive Order, the Health and Human Services Secretary launched the Value- Driven Health Care Initiative, the agenda for which includes four "cornerstones" – transparency of quality information, transparency of pricing information, promotion of health information technology adoption, and creation of incentive mechanisms to promote quality and efficiency. Transparency of pricing will likely foster what is now absent in health care – a price-sensitive consumer. While it is unclear how hospital pricing – and all of its irrational complexity – will be translated for consumer understanding, the net effect may be a flattening of health care pricing, and diminished opportunity for cross-subsidization to cover money-losing procedures and patients. Transparency in both price and quality may, however, boost the market position of specialty hospitals. Specialty hospitals act as "focused factories," serving a subset of patients to perform specific procedures, such as cardiac care and orthopedic surgery.

As such, they focus on delivering well-paying services to an insured pool of patients. Without departments such as emergency, trauma and intensive care, specialty hospitals are free of the regulatory and social obligations that general hospitals are held to. And, with high margins, focused expertise and high volume, specialty hospitals can be very competitive on price and quality. The market and financial advantages of specialty hospitals have not gone unnoticed, and even spurred a moratorium on any new development for awhile. Now that the moratorium has been lifted, the Centers for Medicare & Medicaid (CMS) has proposed correcting inequalities by lowering the reimbursement rate for the diagnostic-related group (DRG) codes that attracted specialty hospital business in the first place. This could be an important leveler since surgery and procedure-related treatment has long been known to attract a higher financial reward than providing medical care, and has therefore created its own set of incentives. This action, though, will not require specialty hospitals to share in providing care that is solely for the public good. Further, it will lower the reimbursement rate that all hospitals receive for performing these same services and further erode future hospital revenue that provides coverage for mission-related services. In the meantime, hospitals are readying for "no pay for preventable events."

As of October 2008, Medicare no longer reimburses hospitals for a growing list of hospital-acquired conditions, such as surgical-site infection and pressure ulcers, as part of its Value-Based Purchasing Initiative. Private-sector payers are quickly following suit. CMS is also looking at ways to equalize payment by using hospital costs rather than charges to set rates. It recently began adjusting payment to better recognize severity of illness and the cost of treating Medicare patients by increasing payments for some services and decreasing payments for others. Fiscal pressures will also keep the pressure on future Medicare and Medicaid provider reimbursements, and it is expected that CMS will continue to seek more avenues to not pay for "preventable conditions" that occur in health care organizations.

BEYOND BORDERS

High health care costs and inadequate access to specialized care are fueling fast growth in medical tourism. Would-be patients in developed countries are traveling thousands of miles – most often to India and Thailand — to receive high-quality care at dramatically lower costs and with no wait. Medical tourism is now a multi-billion-dollar industry. In years past, a medical tourist was someone seeking services that were not covered by health plans, such as cosmetic surgery. Today, a medical tourist is as likely to be seeking full or partial joint replacement, cardiac surgery or even stem cell therapy. Typically, U.S. citizens that have gone abroad have either been uninsured or underinsured and therefore, price-sensitive to the cost of their needed surgeries. The profile of the U.S. medical tourist is changing, however, as selfinsured employers and third-party payers are beginning to add coverage for treatment received abroad as a means to lower their own costs. Rather than wait months or years for an elective surgery, patients in some European countries are crossing borders for more immediate care.

As a result, some European Union (EU) countries, such as the United Kingdom (UK), are reimbursing patients for the cost of acute care received outside of their country of origin on a case-by-case basis. For some European countries, shortening waiting lists may mean exporting patients to elsewhere in the EU, or it may mean importing health care services to bolster the volume of services provided and quicken turnaround times. The phenomenon of the medical tourist seeking complex and necessary care for their well-being outside of their own "health jurisdiction" raises important concerns for the hospital of the future. On one hand, such medical tourism may represent an elaboration of an individual's right to choose.

But, it may also exemplify the failure of a society to fulfill its social contract with its citizens. A global health care marketplace is an increasing competitive threat for U.S. hospitals. A new study from Deloitte finds that the number of patients leaving the U.S. for medical treatment is growing at a faster rate than the number coming for treatment. The study projects that U.S. health care providers will lose nearly $16 billion in revenue this year to outbound medical travel. That figure is expected to grow to $68 billion by 2010, a 325 percent rise. Hospitals are "flattening" for a variety of reasons in addition to globe- trekking patients. The outsourcing of services to offshore entities, such as for radiology, is another way in which hospitals are becoming more global and horizontally configured. But, there are domestic factors that are influencing the flattening of hospitals, as well. Specialty hospitals "disaggregate" hospital services that were once integral to the hospital. In response, hospitals are striking up partnerships with physicians in these ventures so that they can retain some share of the market.

THE HOME TEAM

Despite the impact of globalization and "disaggregation," hospitals have a mission to fulfill to society. No new specialty hospitals or offshore services are being developed to serve the poor, elderly and under- or uninsured. With the coming squeeze on health care pricing and increased competition, hospitals will need to adapt. They will have to learn to do more with less by squeezing out inefficiencies in care delivery. Without the prospect of higher reimbursement rates, hospitals will have to reduce their costs in order to achieve equilibrium in the ratio of payments received to costs expended. There are some seemingly irrational health care expenditures, that on the surface, cry out for a more efficient approach. End-of-life care is an oftmentioned example. In the U.S., highest per capita health care expenditure occurs in the last months of life. Several other countries perform markedly better by this measure and spend less on care at the end of life. However, "to do as they do" is not as easy as it seems.

Differences in social norms, laws, regulations and litigation trends are among the reasons why there are no easy answers to this complex problem. The national focus on health care cost containment strategies and increasingly unstable sources of funding are providing strong influence on hospitals to drive out waste and inefficiencies. Hospitals are increasingly relying on quality improvement tools such as Lean and Six Sigma to create efficient, high-quality care processes. In addition to improved patient safety and higher quality, many organizations are experiencing cost savings through these efforts. For whom these costs are saved remains an issue. Many of the savings, such as those derived from processes that reduce utilization of higher cost services, accrue to health care payers and are revenue losers for hospitals. A realigned and rational payment structure that provides incentives for waste reduction must accompany efforts aimed at creating an efficient – and equally effective – hospital industry. New payment schemes, such as pay-for-performance, are providing hospitals with incentive to focus on specific priorities and maximize quality related to the various measures these programmes track. These programmes will increasingly focus on creating efficiencies in care delivery. But, more alignment of economic incentives with quality goals – such as improved care for the chronically ill — is needed. The key challenge for the hospital of the future is to be able to fulfill its social mission in an environment of constrained federal payment while also investing in new technologies and capital improvements.

TECHNOLOGY FOR THE PROVISION OF CARE

MORE THAN THE BUILDING

- "...no matter what your profession – doctor, lawyer, architect, accountant — ...you better be good at the touchy-feely service stuff, because anything that can be digitized can be outsourced to either the smartest or the cheapest producer, or both... 'Everyone has to focus on what exactly is their value-add.'" — from The World is Flat by Thomas Friedman

With digital technology, radiologists in Bangalore, India do not have to come to the U.S. to practice, U.S. radiology films can go to them. Even more profoundly, digital technology is changing the locus of care delivery and allowing for more care — care that may fall under the umbrella of the hospital — to occur outside of the hospital's walls. In the U.S., the Department of Veterans' Affairs (VA) is on the cutting edge of using digital technology to better meet the needs of a growing number of military veterans, both those who are reaching their senior years and those newly returned from current conflicts.

The VA's national Care Coordination Home Telehealth (CCHT) Programme was first implemented in 2004 to bring about a transition of institutionally based care and chronic care management from hospitals and clinics to patients' own homes when indicated and appropriate. Telehealth applications combined with disease management methods and a comprehensive electronic health record (EHR) support VA care coordinators to remotely monitor patients and thereby enhance and extend care and management. The emphasis of CCHT is on patient self-management and providing a programme of care, rather than the traditional episodic approach to care. Remote monitoring technologies enable disease management questions and objective data – for instance, blood glucose levels of a diabetic patient – to be uploaded to their Electronic Health Record (EHR) daily.

Care coordinators, who are usually nurses and social workers, use these data to prioritize who among their patients needs active care management. CCHT enables a single care coordinator to support a caseload of between 120 and 150 patients depending on case mix. In selected patients, videoconferencing capabilities even allow for virtual physician office visits in the home, which is especially beneficial for patients living in remote areas. This application of technology is not intended to replace the high-touch aspect of care delivery. Because of the heavy emphasis on disease management and vital sign monitoring, CCHT helps to reduce disease complications, and allows patients and caregivers to recognize sooner when a doctor's visit or a hospital admission may be necessary. Currently, the CCHT programme supports the care of 33,883 patients in their own homes. Outcomes data from a cohort of 17,025 patients showed a 20 percent reduction in hospital admissions and a 25 percent reduction in hospital bed days of care. The efficiencies and quality improvements gained through the VA's CCHT programme are helping the VA to serve more patients and change the location of care in accordance with patient preferences.

Veteran patients receiving CCHT care have a mean satisfaction score of 86 percent. CCHT is part of a larger transition in the location of care for patients that is making care more accessible and convenient for veteran patients. In 1995, the VA system had 50,000 hospital beds; today it has 18,000 with the addition of over 1,000 sites of care in local communities that provide primary and ambulatory care. In the intervening period, the VA has become markedly more efficient with a relatively modest increase in clinical staffing, but a dramatic rise in the number of patients served – increasing from 2.5 million to 5 million in the same time frame. Like its counterparts in the non-federal health system, the VA has to do more with less. The migration of care from the hospital bed and physician office to the home that is allowed through technology invites the redefinition of the hospital. Rather than being defined by its number of beds, the "value-add" of the hospital of the future may be its intellectual property. A hospital will be able to lend its expertise to the care of a patient located in a vastly different place than where its facility is located. As an integrated, single-payer system, standardization and innovation is perhaps easier to achieve in the VA system than in hospitals and other health care providers that operate in a more fragmented environment. Implementation of new models of care like the CCHT involve changes in clinical practice, technology infrastructure and business processes. Given the underlying need to care for greater numbers of patients with chronic disease, telehealth and remote patient monitoring could have the same evolutionary impact outside of the VA as it has had within.

MIGHTY I.T.

At the core of the VA's Care Coordination Programme is a comprehensive electronic health record system that is in standard use across VA health delivery sites, including remotely delivered care in the home. In fact, the VA has the largest enterprisewide health information system in the U.S. Outside of the VA, only approximately 11 percent of non-federal hospitals and 12 percent of physician practices have implemented comprehensive electronic health records. Many other countries, including the United Kingdom, Germany, Denmark, Australia and Canada have moved ahead of the U.S. in deploying health information technology. In fact, the U.S. lags a dozen years behind other industrialized countries in health information technology (HIT) adoption. In all of the countries that have implemented national HIT programmes, the costs have been paid by the government and health insurers, and not by the health care providers.

These countries have viewed their investment in HIT as a public good, the benefits of which – reduced costs and improved quality — will mainly accrue to health care payers and patients. Implementation challenges in these countries are also far easier to overcome given their relatively simple payer structures and centralized decision-making capacity as compared to the U.S. With fewer payers – and in some cases, such as in the U.K., centralized vendor selection — the ability to standardize nomenclature and build an interoperable platform is made easier. In the U.S., attempts by payers, coalitions and oversight bodies to influence the rate of adoption of HIT have had mixed results. Following the IOM's release of To Err is Human in 1999, the Leapfrog Group – a consortium of large employers – established its first "leaps" in patient safety for hospitals serving their employees to meet. Among this first set of standards was the requirement that hospitals implement computerized physician order entry (CPOE) systems. Although this requirement came in 2000, still only about five percent of all U.S. hospitals have a CPOE system. Clearly, this leap has fallen short. Leapfrog attributes this to the sheer cost of implementing CPOE and resistance by physicians.

For its part in advancing the adoption of electronic health records, the federal government created the Office of the National Coordinator for Health Information Technology (ONC) within the Department of Health and Human Services (HHS). ONC's primary purpose is to coordinate the development of standards that will allow for interoperability between systems, and a national health information network through which health information can be exchanged. In 2005, HHS created the American Health Information Community (AHIC). This federal advisory committee includes representatives from both the private and public sectors and is charged to provide recommendations to HHS on making health records digital and interoperable, as well as capable of protecting the privacy of patient information. HHS is now in the process of transitioning the AHIC to a successor organization under funding to the Brookings Institution and LMI Consulting. It is envisioned that the AHIC-2 will not start from whole cloth, but will learn from and enhance the work of the existing AHIC's efforts to promote electronic interchange of information.

AHIC-2 is expected to be even more inclusive than AHIC and may also involve some regional loci for its work. In the meantime, HHS has launched demonstration projects through which it provides financial incentives for health care practitioners to use HIT. The Medicare Care Management Demonstration, in part, provides additional payment to physicians who use an EHR certified by the Certification Commission for Health care Information Technology (CCHIT) to electronically submit performance data on 26 measures. The most recent demonstration project allows CMS to make bonus payments to small physician practices that use a certified EHR for clinical documentation and e-prescribing. Payments are determined based on the practices' performance on specific quality measures. It may be that many hospitals still need to be convinced of the value of HIT. While there is a strong evidence base supporting claims that such HIT systems yield significant benefit for the safety and quality of health care, there has been insufficient research conducted to support the return on investment from HIT.

And, the level of required investment can be substantial. Initial implementation costs may range from several hundred thousand dollars for initial implementation in a physician office to millions in a community hospital to tens of millions of dollars in an academic medical center. Annual maintenance of the systems can cost tens of thousands to several million dollars. Many are also wary of the work flow disruptions that a full-scale IT implementation can cause. Enhancing work flow and care process redesign needs to be part and parcel of the implementation plan. Failure to do so can serve to codify already broken or defective care processes. Involving clinical staff who will be using the technology – at the patient's bedside, in the office, pharmacy, lab and home – in its development and providing followon training are key to its success. Issues of interoperability remain generally unsolved as of today.

While health care policymakers and standards bodies hammer out solutions for achieving interoperability of systems that will allow for data sharing between separate entities, many health care providers see this as a reason to wait to invest in HIT.

Unsolved issues around data privacy and fear of system obsolescence further fuel their hesitancy. In the meantime, lack of interoperability between HIT systems and medical devices that have an HIT component –

such as hospital beds that take readings of vital signs but do not integrate with the EHR – slow the workflow of care providers. Indeed, nurses are often the "integrators" of patient information between HIT systems. As new technologies are added to the workplace, it is essential that they be labour-saving in order to conserve already stretched professional resources.

BUY OR BEWARE

With a well-funded biotechnology industry, new technologies are constantly being created with the hope of creating a new disease market or need. This constant barrage of technology purchasing decisions may be difficult to navigate since any new purchase creates an opportunity to increase costs – and waste — in the system. Adding certain new technologies into the health care work place can be very disruptive to work flow and exacerbate inefficiencies. Technologies that are not integrative with other technologies add very little value to the patient's care and the health care worker's practice. With a plethora of cutting-edge information and clinical technology purchasing decisions to be made under a tight budget, health care professionals could use an objective authority to help guide their value-based investments. From 1974-1995, the Congressional Office of Technology Assessment (OTA) provided Congress with objective analysis of contemporary issues involving science and technology.

OTA reports were highly authoritative and well respected. Similar functions in other countries were even modeled after the OTA. But, these reports were sometimes unpopular, especially when their conclusions ran counter to the interests of affected industries. The OTA lost its funding in 1995. The loss of the OTA has left a void. In 2004, a new bill to re-establish some of the capabilities of the OTA was defeated; however, many feel that Congress would benefit from expert analyses of many of the complex scientific and technological issues that are often a source of debate. Though there are private-sector sources for information to support technology decision-making, the OTA served as a public source for much-needed information.

ACHIEVEMENT OF PATIENT-CENTERED CARE

THE MAIN POINT

- At Cincinnati Children's Hospital, family members are included in patient rounds in the pediatric intensive care unit and the hospital encourages family-centered rounds on all of its clinical units. MCG Health System in Augusta, Georgia relies on its Patient and Family Advisory Council to inform the physical design of its care environments and even its compliance with Joint

Commission National Patient Safety Goals. Across its various advisory councils, the University of Washington Medical Center recruits patient and family member volunteers to interview and select residency candidates, and to develop patient educations materials and other supportive programmes for patients and family members. As a result of revelations concerning patient safety, hospitals have had to look inward at practices, policies and even the cultures and attitudes that are prevalent in their delivery settings. In so doing, there is now renewed emphasis and acceptance that it is the patient who is at the center of care. Not only is the patient the main point, but the patient has the greatest stake in their care and as such, should be respected as an equal partner in their care. The elevation of the patient to partner is not a ceremonial title bestowed for a "feel good" moment, but has significant implications for the quality and safety of patient care. When it comes to their health, patients often do not act alone on their own behalf, but their health care decisions are intertwined with those closest to them – their family members or others to whom they are emotionally tied. Family, then, is the third part of the triumvirate in the health care partnership. The Institute for Family-Centered Care defines the core concepts of patient-centered care as: Dignity and Respect – Health care practitioners listen to and honour patient and family perspectives and choices. Patient and family knowledge, values, beliefs and cultural backgrounds are incorporated into the planning and delivery of care.

- *Information Sharing–* Health care practitioners communicate and share complete and unbiased information with patients and families in ways that are affirming and useful. Patients and families receive timely, complete, and accurate information in order to effectively participate in care and decision-making.
- *Participation–* Patients and families are encouraged and supported in participating in care and decision-making at the level they choose.
- *Collaboration–* Patients and families are also included on an institution-wide basis. Health care leaders collaborate with patients and families in policy and programme development, implementation, and evaluation; in health care facility design; and in professional education, as well as in the delivery of care.

Another resource for patient-centered care guidance is Planetree. Planetree is a non-profit organization that provides education and information to health care organizations to facilitate the delivery of patient-centered care. Planetree's Patient-Centered Care Designation Programme recognizes hospitals that meet its criteria for patient-centered care. These criteria have been compiled based upon the experiences of hospitals who have achieved patient-centered care, as well as the feedback of patients. The criteria are used to measure organizations' structures and functions that support patient-centered care concepts; human interactions; patient education and community access to information; family involvement; nutrition; the architecture and interior design of the healing environment; art programmes; spirituality and diversity; integrative therapies; community health; and measurement.

NOTHING WITHOUT ME

Engaging patients in their care has real implications for the quality and safety of patient care. A large study of adult patients with chronic or serious conditions who were engaged in a collaborative care model had better control of their blood pressure, blood glucose levels, and serum cholesterol than patients who had less confidence either in their doctors or their ability to care for themselves. Another study of patients hospitalized for acute myocardial infarction found that patients who rated hospitals poorly on Picker Institute measures of patient-centered care had poorer health outcomes than those who experienced more patient-centered care. The experiences of MCG Health System in Augusta, Georgia attests to the prospects for patient-centered care in improving quality and safety. In 2003, the health system redesigned its intensive care unit for neuroscience patients to allow patients' families to stay with them at all times. The observances of family members were valued by the unit's clinical staff.

Owing to these insights and improved communications, medication errors in the unit decreased 62 percent, length of stay decreased 50 percent, and the staff vacancy rate fell from 7.5 percent to zero. Patient satisfaction ratings increased from the tenth percentile to the 95th. In the words of an MCG staff member, the families "helped us help their loved ones." Engagement of patients and families empowers patients to participate in care decisions, provide self-care, and protect themselves from potential harm. In fact, The Joint Commission's National Patient Safety Goal 13 specifically requires health care organization staff to encourage patients' active involvement in their care as a patient safety strategy. Goal 13 further requires staff to identify ways in which the patient and his or her family can report concerns about safety and encourage them to do so. The rationale for this goal states that "communication with the patient and family about all aspects of care, treatment, and services is an important characteristic of a culture of safety. When the patient knows what to expect, he or she is more aware of possible errors and choices. The patient can also be an important source of information about potential adverse events and hazardous conditions." The aspect of patient empowerment within patient-centered care has led to the notion of "nothing about me, without me."

MOMENTUM

In addition to Joint Commission standards and safety goals, other organizational and professional accrediting bodies increasingly emphasize the importance of engaging patients in the delivery of care. In the U.S., the inclusion of information pertaining to patients' perspectives of care on the CMS Web site, Hospital Compare, provides a powerful incentive for hospitals to better meet the expectations of patients. The survey – called H-CAHPS – addresses issues such as the quality of nurse and physician communications with patients, discharge instructions, and medication education. In the international arena, the U.K. National Health Service (NHS) is requiring its hospitals and primary care clinics to engage patients and family in quality improvement efforts. Across Canada, patients are being similarly engaged.

The World Health Organization (WHO) has also made patient and family engagement in patient safety improvement a major priority of its World Alliance for Patient Safety, launched in 2004. Patients and families are also driving momentum. Several patient advocacy organizations, such as Partnerships for Patient Safety (p4ps) and PULSE are organized around the goal of advancing patient-centered care and improving patient safety. Social momentum for patient-centered care is also likely to increase with the growth of consumerdirected health plans and health savings accounts (HSAs). Such health plans increase the health care consumers' responsibility for making value-based health care purchasing decisions. Technology is another momentum-building factor. The advent of personal health records (PHRs) will provide patients with "point and click" access to their own health records as well as enhanced communications capabilities with their care providers. Technology that is allowing patients to receive higher levels of care in their homes underscores the need for a patient-centered approach to care, especially as their role as "partner" in care delivery becomes a 24/7 endeavor. These patients and families need personalized education and training, as well as a professional support system so that the transition to home-based care is safe and effective for all involved.

CUSTOM AND CULTURE

While momentum is certainly building and the concept of patient-centered care is widely embraced, much is still getting lost in the execution. There are barriers, not the least of which is the heightened need for patient education when practitioners seemingly have less time to spend with patients – ala the 10-minute office visit. There are also issues of health literacy – in the U.S. alone, nearly half the population lacks the skills necessary to obtain, process, and understand basic health information and services needed to make appropriate health decisions. The focus in patient-centered care on transparency can make hospital risk managers uneasy. Yet, several studies have revealed that what patients really want – open disclosure, communications and collaboration – nurtures, rather than harms, patient and caregiver relationships. It is also important to underscore what patient-centered care is not. In some countries, the term is a euphemism for a lower tier of care, where the de facto caregiver is the family – not in partnership with practitioners – but on their own.

There are other cultural differences to patient-centered care. In Thai culture, the family will stay at the patient's bedside round-the-clock and help with feeding and personal support. But, neither a Thai patient nor family member will generally participate in decision- making — that is the province of the physician, whose level of education is held in high esteem. In any country, it is also important to recognize that not every patient wants to be a partner in their care, nor do they wish their family to be. The level of partnership may vary – some patients may wish to be 50/50 partners, others may wish for much less. For the hospital of the future, care must be increasingly customized to the personal expectations, cultural beliefs and traditions, and language needs of the patient. In eliciting patients' needs and expectations of their care, hospitals may need to perform an intake interview that covers these topics at the time of admission. Instilling patient-centered care is not just about changing policies and practices; it is about changing culture, which is never easily done. For staff to be empathetic to patients, the hospital must also have an empathetic culture for staff. Staff members need to be supported through systems that protect them from harm – and from doing harm. In the absence of such cultures and work environments, staff members may become overburdened and increasingly demoralized. To achieve a culture that is patient-centered and supportive of staff, hospital leadership and staff must share common beliefs and values. Coming to these common beliefs and values may be the hardest part of achieving cultural change.

SERVING THE UNDERSERVED

In the U.S., there are specific populations who are the least likely to receive patient-centered care. For minority groups and the poor, disparities in health care quality and access persist. The 2007 National Health care Disparities Report issued by the Agency for Health care Research and Quality reveals that, overall, disparities have not been reduced despite the growing body of evidence of their existence, though there have been small gains. Positive examples include the adequacy of hemodialysis for Black and for White patients, and the hospital admission rate among Hispanics and the poor and their White, affluent counterparts for perforated appendix.

These small gains are offset by the persistence of wide disparities in health care quality that have resulted in disproportionate numbers of minorities and poor who have AIDS, lower immunization rates, and lack access to prenatal care, among other examples of unequal treatment. Sometimes it is the provenance of their illness that creates disparate access to quality health care for patients. Mentally ill patients are perhaps the most underserved patient population today. A report from a special commission to President Bush claims that half of Americans who need mental health care are not getting it, even if they have sought it. Mainly due to a payment system that does not support the provision of psychiatric care, many hospital- based and free-standing psychiatric services have closed or reduced their number of beds. In fact, from 1995 to 1999, the number of psychiatric beds in this country shrunk by 38 percent. All the while, demand for inpatient psychiatric care has climbed, leaving the mentally ill often with nowhere else to turn but to the hospital emergency department for care.

In fact, emergency departments across the country report an influx of mentally ill patients coming through their doors. With so few alternatives to place these patients in a psychiatric bed, the emergency department often holds these patients for hours, even days. Though the roots of the problem began more than a decade ago, it is a problem that worsens year to year. In a 2007 AHA survey, 42 percent of hospitals reported an increase in boarding behavioral health patients in the emergency department. The boarding of psychiatric patients brings its own particular strain and costs. Crowded emergency departments, with staff and resources stretched thin, cannot provide the intense care and monitoring psychiatric patients in crisis need, which is best provided in an appropriate setting and by specially trained health care workers.

ON THE RISE

Today, half of all hospitalized patients have one or more chronic condition, such as diabetes, heart disease and asthma. The prevalence of chronic illness is expected to steadily increase. By 2030, it is estimated that 171 million people will have at least one chronic illness. By this same year, older adults will account for more than 20 percent of the population. While older adults are expected to live longer, this will not be without personal health challenges. More than 75 percent of adults over age 65 suffer from at least one chronic condition, and many have multiple conditions. Among current Medicare beneficiaries, 20 percent have five or more chronic conditions. Aging is not the only factor driving the burgeoning ranks of the chronically ill. Owing to its significantly higher rates of obesity and smoking, the U.S. has a significantly higher rate of associated diseases – such as diabetes, hypertension and heart disease – than European countries. According to the Centers for Disease Control and Prevention (CDC), 80 percent of diabetes, heart disease and stroke could be eliminated through reductions in smoking and obesity. There is widespread recognition that care for the chronically ill in the U.S. is falling short. An oftcited report from RAND indicates that the chronically ill receive approximately half of recommended care.

At the root of this issue is the predominant organization of the health delivery and payment system to support the diagnosis and treatment of acute, or episodic, conditions. Patients with chronic illness, especially those with multiple conditions, often receive care from multiple providers and take many medications. Because this care is uncoordinated, patients may experience duplicative services and testing, avoidable hospitalization, and adverse drug events. As a result, care is often fragmented, ineffective and costly for people with chronic diseases. Optimal care for people with chronic diseases involves coordinated, continuous treatment by a multidisciplinary team of health care professionals. These patients need education and tools to support self- management, and connections to community resources for their social, mental health and home health needs. For the hospital of the future, providing patientcentered care means better meeting the needs of all of its patients, including the underserved, the aged and the chronically ill who will fill its beds in greater numbers.

PATIENT-CENTERED TRANSFORMATION

To increase their reliability in delivering patientcentered care, hospitals can turn to the process improvement tools — such as Six Sigma and Lean, among others — that have proved effective for transforming other industries. A glimpse of that transformation can be seen at hospitals like Virginia Mason Medical Center in Seattle, which has applied these tools to improve the quality of care for patients with low back pain and other conditions, increase adherence to evidence-based care, and decrease costs. In ThedaCare hospitals in southern Wisconsin, application of these methods to general medical units has allowed the hospitals to reduce medication errors, the average amount of time these patients are hospitalized, and the fees charged for certain procedures. New York- Presbyterian Hospital used these tools to reduce average length of stay for patients undergoing cardiac and orthopedic procedures, reduce medication errors and patient falls, and increase patient satisfaction rates.

THE STAFFING CHALLENGE

WIDE AND DEEP

Hospitals rank second as a source of private-sector jobs nationwide. In urban areas, hospitals are among the top ten employers, and are often the largest employer in rural areas. Health care, broadly, contributed more jobs to the economy than any other industry in the last several years. Still, the demand for certain health professionals outstrips supply. Workforce shortages have persistently plagued hospitals over the last several years. In 2007, as well as in previous years, it has ranked in the top five issues confronting hospital CEOs according to a poll conducted by the American College of Health care Executives. Staffing problems are widespread across health care professions.

Therapists – physical, occupational and speech – are in especially short supply and increasingly difficult to recruit from year to year. Vacancy rates for these positions exceeded 11 percent by year-end 2006. Registered nurses, pharmacists, nursing assistants, licensed practical nurses, and laboratory and imaging technicians all have vacancy rates in the range of six percent for technicians to eight percent for RNs. There is also growing national concern over shortages of physicians – already a problem in several states – that is expected to worsen as demand outstrips supply. By 2020, the U.S. may be short 85,000 physicians. It is not just the frontline clinicians that are difficult to hire and retain. Hospital executive positions have high turnover. As many as half of nurse executives, and 14 to 18 percent of chief executive officers, will leave their jobs in a year. Pervasive staffing problems challenge the ability of the hospital to perform its most fundamental functions. Studies show that there is an association between registered nurse staffing and hospitalrelat- ed mortality, failure to rescue, and higher risk of complications, among other negative patient outcomes.

In addition, beds that are not staffed cannot be filled by patients, undermining the admissions process, especially admissions from the emergency department (ED). Nearly half of all hospital emergency departments report being at or over capacity, and the majority of urban hospitals experience time on diversion – when they are closed to incoming ambulances. The primary reason for going on diversion is a lack of staffed critical care beds. Staffing shortages, overall, are among the top five conditions that lead to ambulance diversion. In addition to ED overcrowding and diversion, about half of hospitals report that staffing shortages contribute to decreased staff satisfaction. Decreased patient satisfaction, reduced numbers of staffed beds, increased length of stay, increased wait times for surgery, as well as cancelled surgeries also follow in the wake of staffing shortages. Low staff satisfaction is a persistent problem for many hospitals. Hospital-based nurses, for instance, have job dissatisfaction rates that are three to four times higher than the average U.S. worker. Low dissatisfaction rates among nurses is not an American phenomenon, but occurs in other countries where it has been studied, such as Canada, England and Scotland. Yet, the sentiment is not universal. Nurses employed in facilities that have been awarded Magnet Recognition® from the American Nurses Credentialing Center (ANCC) report being more satisfied with their work. In addition to higher staff satisfaction, Magnet status strengthens nursing recruitment and retention efforts. Independent studies show that patients in Magnet hospitals have shorter lengths of stay, lower mortality rates and higher satisfaction, and benefit from a richer staff mix.

A GLOBAL PREDICAMENT

As perhaps the most in-demand health care resource across the globe, plenty of nurses are being "insourced" into other countries. The U.S. has long depended on migrating nurses to fill its growing gap between nurse supply and demand. This practice also occurs in other highly developed countries, at the expense of the less developed, where many migrating nurses originate. Nurses are not the only migrating health care worker. Physicians, pharmacists and lab technicians are on the move as well. The WHO reports that the situation of migrating workers is most desperate in poor countries and continents. Africa, for instance, holds 11 percent of the world's population, but it hosts 25 percent of the disease burden, and yet, it employs three percent of all health care workers.

Twenty-five percent of African-trained doctors work in wealthy Organisation for Economic Co-operation and Development (OECD) countries. In Ghana, 40 physicians graduated in 2004 from the government-financed medical education system, but only two remained in the country. The others left for either the U.S. or U.K. to practice. The shortage of health care workers is exacerbating the devastation wrought by the AIDS crisis in Africa. According to the WHO, because of the shortage of health care workers at least 1.3 billion people around the world have no access to basic health care services. In response, the WHO is pressing countries across the globe to address the ethical and financial impacts of worker migration, as well as efforts to retain workers within their country of origin. The practice of health care worker importation and exportation is, of course, unsustainable. But, it begs the question: Who will staff the hospital of the future?

STOPS AND STARTS

In the U.S., a poor economy is driving people back to work and providing some optimism for a more robust nursing workforce. New research finds that after a net loss of more than 10,500 nurses in 2004 and 2005, health care gained roughly 18,700 nurses in 2006. In 2007, the industry added 84,200 nurses despite a drop in real wages. Current projections for the shortage of nurses in the U.S. puts the number at 340,000 by 2020, which is significantly fewer than previous projections of 760,000.

An important distinction of the evolving shortage is that the nurses who have stepped forward to help fill the gap are markedly older – in their late twenties and early thirties – whereas the number of new entries in their early to mid-twenties is at the lowest level in 40 years. As the average age of the nurse moves upward, there are implications for hospital design and ergonomics that are needed to support the health and longevity of the nurse on the job. During the first year on the job, the average voluntary turnover rate of new hospital nurses is 27 percent. This likely reflects the combination of inadequate educational preparation of the nurse for the realities of practice, as well as longstanding work environment issues that have contributed to low satisfaction rates of hospital-employed nurses. Among these issues are long shifts and persistent fatigue; lack of leadership that empowers nursing staff; unavailability of supportive technologies; and lack of innovation in redesigning and improving the role and workflow of the nurse. A recent time and motion study to determine how medical-surgical nurses spend their time found that nearly three-quarters of nurses' time was spent on documentation, medication administration and care coordination, but only one-fifth of their time was spent on direct patient care.

Further, nurses walked between one mile and five miles every shift in an effort to "hunt and gather" needed supplies or information. The inordinate amount of time spent on documentation – almost one-third of all of their time – points to the need to examine the role of the nurse and its inherent processes. Few nurses would cite "paperwork," as necessary as it is, as the reason they chose nursing as their profession. A major bottleneck in efforts to add new nurses to the workforce remains a lack of capacity at the educational level. According to data from the American Association of Colleges of Nursing (AACN), enrollment in entry-level baccalaureate nursing programmes increased by almost five percent from 2006 to 2007. While this increase represents a positive enrollment trend over the past several years, more than 30,000 qualified applicants were denied entry into baccalaureate nursing programmes in 2007 due primarily to an intensifying shortage of nurse faculty. The gap between supply and demand in the nursing workforce will be difficult to fill without resolution of the crisis in nursing education capacity.

HIGH TOUCH, HIGH TECH

As patients' needs and health care delivery become ever-more complex, it is difficult for clinicians to keep pace. Hospitalized patients have higher acuity and are more likely to have comorbidities, while hospital stays have shortened. Average length-ofstay for hospitalized patients has declined by 25 percent since the 1980s. Since the late 1990s, the Food and Drug Administration (FDA) has approved more than 500,000 new medical devices. At the same time, ever-increasing developments in pharmaceuticals, biologics and genomics are expanding the knowledge demands of practitioners. While many advances in technology help to improve patient outcomes, the sheer volume of technologies and the attendant knowledge required has made health care delivery vastly more complex. Additionally, new technologies often provide new, sometimes unforeseen, opportunities for error. The impact of this developing complexity weighs heavily on the hospital-based clinician. One way in which the nursing profession has responded is by the creation of the Clinical Nurse Leader™ role. The American Association of Colleges of Nursing (AACN) has developed this new nursing role to better prepare nurses for clinical leadership in all health care settings.

These masters'-prepared nurses are expected to be direct caregivers, managing the care of patients within clinical microsystems. The Clinical Nurse Leader™ certification process ensures that these nurses bring evidencebased practices to care settings and are able to apply quality improvement principles to the measurement, assessment and improvement of patientcare outcomes. According to the AACN, currently about 60 colleges and universities offer the master's degree programme that prepares the Clinical Nurse Leader.™ Scientific progress, such as new developments in biologics, genomics, robotic preparation and automated distribution, is affecting the level of technologic expertise that the hospital pharmacist must have. In fact, the profession raised the entry-level degree for a pharmacist to a doctorate (Pharm.D) to ensure a better-prepared pharmacist workforce. Many pharmacists who practice in hospitals also complete residency training.

The downside of this higher standard is that it created a roadblock for the entry of new pharmacy students. Indeed, hospitals surveyed by the AHA reported an eight percent vacancy rate for pharmacists at the end of 2006. The role of the hospital pharmacist is expected to change as well. Always a valued member of the health care team, the role of the pharmacist is likely to become more visible in patient-centered care delivery as a way to combat the high volume of medication errors that occur in the hospital setting. As hospital pharmacists become more involved in direct patient care, there is a requisite need to accommodate new learning in the education and training of pharmacy students. There are concerns that hospitals and health systems may not have the capacity to accommodate the growing numbers of pharmacy students who will require this experiential education. The involvement of pharmacists in direct patient care has also resulted in a greater reliance on trained and certified pharmacy technicians, who assist with the preparation and delivery of medications.

A.CHANGING OF THE GUARD

A changing of the guard has been occurring in hospitals over the last several years, a change that is likely to become the standard in hospitals of the future. Hospitalists – physicians who practice primarily hospital-base care – have been increasingly staffing U.S. hospitals. It is estimated that by 2010, 30,000 hospitalists will be staffing U.S. hospitals. As hospitalists are gaining prevalence, the concept is also expanding from general practice and internal medicine to include medical and surgical specialists. The recent growth of the hospitalist movement in the U.S. can be attributed to a number of factors. Fewer office-based primary care physicians choose to provide hospital-based care. Work hours for residents, who have traditionally provided 24/7 hospital care, have been reduced in recent years. Hospitalists fill these gaps by providing acute care expertise to patients throughout their hospital stay. A recent study in the New England Journal of Medicine found that patients cared for by hospitalists have average lengths of stay in the hospital and associated costs that are slightly reduced.

TEAM-BASED CARE

With staffing shortages still looming in the hospital of the future, hospitals may need to accomplish more with fewer health professionals. Well functioning teams can get more done than any one individual. Teamwork also has a significantly positive impact on the safety of health care delivery. Studies show that well functioning teams make fewer mistakes than do individuals. Acquisition of team skills does not occur by happenstance. Health professionals must be educated and trained to value and demonstrate desired team behaviours. To that end, knowledge of teamwork components and the competencies required to effectively participate as team members should be introduced early in health care professional education and fostered throughout professional training and continuing education. Further, teamwork skills, knowledge and performance should be incorporated into the oversight and assessment of health professionals and organizations in order to ensure and sustain its widespread adoption.

Both classroom and simulator-based methodologies can be used for team training. In addition to team skills, members of the care-giving team must have the requisite knowledge and skills to effectively care for older adults and the chronically ill. Today, older adults account for 35 percent of all hospital stays, 26 percent of all physician visits, and 34 percent of all prescriptions. Yet, less than one percent of registered nurses and pharmacists are certified in geriatrics. While more than 7,000 physicians are currently certified in geriatrics, the need is much greater. By 2030, it is estimated that 36,000 geriatricians will be needed to care for the burgeoning population of older adults. As the number of older adults and patients with one more chronic illness rises, so too, must the competencies of those who provide their care. Hospitals play a key role in fostering the competence of all health care workers in caring for geriatric patients. Hospitals must also increase the recruitment and retention of geriatric specialists and caregivers.

Team-based care models may be expanded and bolstered by the potential payment model advocated by the Medicare Payment Advisory Commission (MedPAC). MedPAC recommends a bundled Medicare payment approach, under which physicians and hospitals receive a fixed payment for a select set of episodes of care. An episode is defined as the hospital stay plus 30 days after discharge. Today, physicians and hospitals are paid separately under different payment schemes by CMS for hospital-based care. A bundled approach, it is believed, will reduce variation in costs and quality and encourage joint accountability. This concept will be tested by CMS beginning in January 2009 with its Acute Care Episode (ACE) demonstration, which will offer bundled payment for 28 cardiac and nine orthopedic inpatient surgical services in four states. Among the many expectations for bundled payment is that it will influence physicians and hospitals to closely integrate their services, which will be necessary in order to accept bundled payments.

DESIGN OF THE PHYSICAL ENVIRONMENT

SAFE BY DESIGN

Though the recent economic downturn and a tightened credit market has slowed hospital construction in the U.S., there has been a remarkable hospital building boom underway fueled by increasing demand for health care services and increasingly obsolete hospital plants. In 2007, $35.4 billion in health care construction projects were completed, more than a $10 billion increase from the previous year. Projections foresee the health care industry among the only bright points for construction in the next couple of years. This investment offers the opportunity to remake the hospital — its design, culture and practices – to better meet the needs of patients and families and the aspirations of those that provide their care.

Building more of the same will freeze into place persistent problems with which hospitals must already contend — such as unsafe care, hospitalacquired infection, and worker fatigue – that otherwise could be mitigated through the application of evidence-based design. Several hundred studies have revealed hospital design characteristics that work for improving patient safety and health care outcomes, and providing a supportive environment for hospital staff. Yet, most new hospitals are not being built "safe by design." New hospitals will increasingly care for more elderly patients. And, as more care moves out to ambulatory and home settings, hospitalized patients will be the sickest and most vulnerable. More than ever, hospitals will need to be designed to safely accommodate these fragile patients. Prominent threats to patient safety – medication errors, patient falls, and errors made during patient transfers, among them – can be mitigated through evidence-based design. Better lighting and reduced noise levels can help avoid distractions that often lead to caregiver errors in the medication process.

Decentralized nursing stations allow nurses to better see and hear the patients under their care and observe changes in skin colour and breathing, as well as to prevent falls that occur when a patient is unobserved. Rooms that are designed for the patient bed and bathroom entrance to be seen from the hallway also enhance observation. Multiacuity beds that reduce the number of transfers, or "hand-offs," of patients from one unit to another, in turn, reduce the opportunity for errors to occur. The regulatory infrastructure can stifle design innovations meant to reduce the risk of patient injury. Though multi- acuity beds that allow a patient to remain in the same bed while their care level is stepped down from critical care to medical-surgical nursing may make sense, in some states they do not meet state licensure stipulations regarding patient bed designations and thereby are disqualified for reimbursement. Single-patient rooms may have the single most important impact on patient safety. In addition to enhancing patient privacy, allowing for confidential discussions and accommodating family members, single rooms help protect patients' health. Spread of infection is a daily risk in every of hospital. When patients are isolated from one another, there are fewer chances for microbes to be spread.

In addition to patient-to-patient spread, caregiverto- patient spread is common. Well-placed sinks and alcohol gel dispensers can prompt caregivers to wash their hands, which is an essential part of any infection control programme. Single rooms further improve the rate of hand-washing when crossing the barriers between patient rooms prompts caregivers to wash their hands. Whereas, in a double patient room, the transition from one patient to the next is quick and barrier-free; too little time to stop and think about hand- washing. Single rooms also allow for better air quality management and can be more thoroughly decontaminated between occupancies.

FLAT WORLD PHENOMENA

Infection control, always a high priority for any hospital, becomes paramount in the face of a potential global epidemic. Emergency preparedness is a key priority to be addressed in the design of the hospital of the future. In today's ever-flattening world, individuals are more globalized – they travel more, both virtually and in person. The supply chain is also more globalized and could easily be disrupted by a global epidemic: "… when the world is flattening – when some 80 percent of the raw materials that go into pharmaceutical drugs sold in America come from overseas suppliers, and when the rubber that keeps surgical masks tight on your face comes through a just- in-time supply chain that starts in Indonesia or Africa, stretches through Europe, and then skips over to America – our ability to cope with any pandemic would be sharply reduced."

Thanks to the ubiquity of airline travel, an infectious disease can move quickly in a flat world. Once SARS appeared in rural China, it spread to five countries within 24 hours. In a matter of months, it had spread to 30 countries on six continents. With the SARS epidemic, hospitals that were sought for care became the vectors for SARS transmission. Open bay intensive care units (ICUs), public waiting areas, and emergency departments all became central stations for contracting SARS. Tuberculosis has also been known to be similarly spread. The good news is that hospitals can be designed to mitigate these risks. The transformation of the physical environment of care must also take into consideration future needs such as achieving surge capacity in response to disaster.

STANDARDIZED FLEXIBILITY

- Standardization reduces complexity, which is important when flexibility is needed, as is the case for increasing surge capacity. Importantly, standardization is a key strategy in human factors design as a means to reduce the risk of error and improve quality. Human factors design focuses on improving the human-system interface by designing better systems and processes. For hospitals, standardization of patient rooms, treatment rooms, equipment and care processes, reduces reliance on short-term memory. In room design, standardizing details such as the location of bed controls, light switches, and even, which cupboards store latex gloves, for instance, are important considerations for optimizing the human- system interface. The lengthy cycle of design and construction is often overtaken by the rapid cycle of innovation in medicine and technology. As a result, some buildings are partially obsolete when they open, and nearly every health care structure will be obsolete in some way before it has completed its useful life. Design for flexibility is a way to reduce the inconvenience and cost of these inevitable disruptions. Master planning strategies: Every design should have planned zones for future growth. These can appear as a dotted line on the site plan, or may be developed as constructed but unoccupied shell space, or as structural capacity to allow for future vertical additions to a building.
- Loose-fit design: Many designs make an effort to design precisely to the absolute minimum square footage justified by the programme of space requirements, yet such designs are the first to reveal difficulties when new programmes appear, or existing programmes grow or shrink. The concept of loose-fit is to design with larger spaces that can be used for more than the minimum function originally proposed, and to arrange them in departments or groupings that allow for future adjustments.
- Adaptable flexibility: Spaces can be designed to adapt to multiple uses. An example is a patient room that can be adapted for the purpose of simple procedures such as a line insertion. The different function can be accommodated by simply adapting the space because it has been planned to serve a range of possibilities.
- Convertible flexibility: Another type of flexibility is when, with relatively low effort, time, and/or cost, a space can be converted to another use. Examples of this type of flexibility include a storage space with a knockout panel in the slab to allow for a future elevator, or a patient room with plumbing, gasses, and electrical systems in the wall for future conversion to critical care.

- Robust utilities: In order to offer flexibility in design, the utility and communication infrastructure of a health care facility should be capable of expansion and upgrade. Availability of utility and network capacity simplifies and dramatically reduces the cost of future projects.
- Plug-and-play infrastructure: Just as all the utilities of the city are uninterrupted when one property undergoes a construction or demolition project, a hospital should be designed so that the utility and primary horizontal and vertical circulation infrastructure remains in service while departments, wings, or entire buildings are added or removed.

PLACE OF WORK

In addition to protecting patients, hospital design is integral to protecting hospital workers and enhancing the work they do. About one-third of a nurse's time on shift is spent walking. Not only is this time spent walking between the centralized nursing station and patient rooms, but on hunting and gathering various supplies.

Decentralizing nursing stations and supplies – bringing both closer to the patients – would reduce wasted time and fatigue. Other physical stressors include noise, that when reduced, as previously mentioned, results in less fatigue and reduced risk of error. A great deal of heavy lifting, turning, and transporting patients goes on in hospitals that could be alleviated by proper hoists and other ergonomic technologies. Involving staff in the design process is essential for creating a physical environment that improves work flow. In the future, the application of design improvements to time-consuming nursing tasks, such as medication administration and documentation, may yield new gains in efficiency.

As pharmacists increasingly counsel patients on drugs and therapeutic regimens, the physical environment of the pharmacy must be made to accommodate these confidential discussions. New design concepts have been shown to give hospital clinical staff more time to spend with patients, while also allowing the hospital to expand its capacity to treat patients. Designing a hospital with safety in mind helps to create a safety culture. Involving patients and families, in addition to staff, in the design of the physical environment also helps to assure the patientcenteredness of the organizational culture. The culture of the workplace can be transformed by the physical demonstration that the organization embraces patient and staff safety, and collegial health care delivery.

BEING GREEN

Global climate change and harm wrought from chemical contamination are no longer speculative. In congruence with their mission, hospitals in the future must be healthy places to be in and live near. In 1996, the Environmental Protection Agency (EPA) declared medical waste incineration to be the greatest source of dioxin contamination in the atmosphere. At that time, there were 5,000 medical waste incinerators. Today there are fewer than 100 still in operation. That momentum needs to continue and be broadened to include the elimination of toxic materials used inside the hospital. The chemical compound polyvinyl chloride (PVC) is ubiquitous in the hospital environment. It is used in I.V. and blood bags, plastic tubing and an array of other medical supplies. When PVCbased products, such as nasogastric tubes, are used invasively, they can leach toxic chemicals that enter the body.

One of these chemicals has proven to be a reproductive toxicant, which led the National Toxicology Programme to declare that infants in hospitals are at risk from this chemical. PVC, which is also commonly used in hospital building materials, emits toxins into the air, putting patients and staff at risk. Interior exposure to PVC has been definitively linked to asthma. With the prevalence of PVC exposure, as well as exposure to other noxious chemicals such as cleaning agents and pesticides, it is no wonder that poor air quality is the most frequent cause of work-related asthma in health care workers. Hospitals are huge consumers of energy – natural gas and electricity — second only to the food-service industry in energy consumption. The costs of such energy consumption will increasingly comprise an unaffordable portion of the hospital budget. These costs plus growing concern over global warming are influencing hospitals to use cleaner, more efficient sources of energy and to reduce their global footprint.

Accordingly, hospitals will need to use fewer resources and produce less waste. One hundred U.S. hospitals are finding it easier to be green by piloting the Green Guide for Health Care (GGHC), standards modeled on those of the U.S. Green Building Council's Leadership in Energy and Environmental Design (LEED), in their construction projects. The GGHC standards actually exceed LEED standards and align environmental health considerations with health system priorities. The GGHC has received strong endorsement – Kaiser Permanente has committed to using it for building projects across its system, and the City of Boston is recommending it to city hospitals that are embarking on expansion plans. A healthy hospital environment also extends to the food that is served in that environment. Food that is served in hospitals should promote and not undermine health. Large health care systems, such as Kaiser Permanente and Catholic Health care West, have led the way in implementing policies that require healthy food choices for patients and also support sustainable farming practices – food production that is local, humane and environmentally protective.

CONCLUSION

A century ago, people advocated for hospitals to be less institutional and impersonal in their approach to patient care. They worried about neglect of the aged and the chronically ill. The vision was expressed for a system of care, led by hospitals, which encompassed patients' family and social needs. People foresaw the need for hospital care to migrate from within the hospital's four walls, out into the community, even into the home. Everything old is new again. The increasing prevalence of chronic illness among patients served by hospitals and an aging population should compel hospitals to pursue models of care that would best meet the needs of patients across the care continuum, wherever those services are delivered. In this, hospitals are ideally positioned to lead efforts to create a true "system" of care delivery. In hospitals that embrace the concepts of patientcentered care and support the development of their workforce, no one should be neglected.

The application of digital technologies is already extending the reach of hospital care into the community and into the home. The hospital of the future may one day be defined by its intellectual property, rather than its physical facility. That said, the physical design of the hospital has significant implications for the ability of the hospital to meet its goals for care that is safe, patient-centered, clinically effective and collaboratively delivered. It also represents the physical manifestation of the hospital's commitment to environmental health and sustainability. There are factors that will be — to lesser and greater extents — out of the hospital's control as the future unfolds. Fair and rational payment strategies that align with national quality goals can be advocated for, but they cannot be assured. In the meantime, hospitals must do their part to reduce error and waste, and increase efficiencies as a means of improving safety and containing costs. The principles put forth here are meant to guide the hospitals to be better prepared to accomplish what is being asked of them.

❐

Chapter - 7

Public Interference in Health Industry

WHY THE PUBLIC ROLE IN HEALTH CARE MATTERS

Health care in about 1990 cost at least $1.7 trillion, or about 8 per cent of world income, making it one of the largest industries in the global economy. On average, 60 per cent of this is public spending. If this spending is excessive or otherwise inappropriate, the consequences for the economy and for health outcomes could be substantial.

Governments also provide a large share of health services, sometimes as large as the share in spending, and often intervene in various ways in the private health care market. Since most health care is a private good, it is surprising that so much of it is provided, financed or regulated by the state. In contrast to what happens in many other sectors of the economy, this substantial public role is most pronounced in high income countries which are generally very market-oriented; the state usually finances a smaller share of health care in poorer countries.

Does this pattern provide models for the future development of the health sector and the public role in it, for lowincome countries? And is the variation among countries in the amount and kind of public intervention associated with differences in people's health, in what is spent on health care or in how well health systems function?

Besides consuming large resources, many health systems are regarded as inefficient or inequitable or both; they are often described as in "crisis", as needing "reform", or as having "failed". Are the supposed failures of health systems real? If so, they might be caused by misguided public intervention, so they could be corrected by a smaller or different public role and a greater reliance on private markets. Or governments might intervene for sound reasons, to correct or compensate for failings in those markets; that is, outcomes would be even worse if left entirely to the private sector. Is there an appropriate frontier between private and public action, and a best combination of instruments for the state to use when it intervenes? These and related questions must be confronted in any reform effort. It is relatively simple to conclude that governments should do certain things and should leave others to private activity; but often there is a variety of possible solutions and no obviously best approach. Theory does not always provide clear answers, and the empirical evidence is incomplete, extremely varied and difficult to interpret.

CHOICES FOR STATE INTERVENTION

It matters not only whether governments intervene, but also how they do it: the second essential question is what the public sector should do, given that some problem in the private market appears to warrant some public action. This is particularly important because government failings in the health sector are also common, and often result from intervening in the wrong ways or with the wrong instruments.

There are five distinct instruments of public intervention: arranged from the least to the greatest intrusion into private decisions, these are to:

1. Inform, which may mean to persuade, but does not require anyone to do anything. Governments do this when they publicize the health risks of smoking, or include health and basic hygiene education in public schools. These are examples of information directed at consumers, but governments also inform health care providers and suppliers of health care inputs, as by conducting research and disseminating information on disease patterns and on the effects and risks of medical procedures.
2. Regulate, which determines how a private activity may be undertaken. Governments sometimes regulate the medical profession by setting standards for doctors or accrediting hospitals, although these activities may also be undertaken by private bodies. And government regulation is common in the insurance industry, in the importation of medical equipment, drugs and supplies and in the protection of food and water quality. More generally, governments can influence private health care activity in many ways, often combining regulation with some financial incentives to offset the costs but without public financing. Regulation is usually pursuant to a law, and is often determined by an executive or administrative body.

3. Mandate, which obligates someone to do something and to pay for it. Compliance with regulations can also imply substantial private costs; but a mandated activity is different in that it must be performed, whereas a private producer can react to regulation by choosing not to undertake the activity. Mandates are usually specified in law, which may subsequently be adumbrated by regulation. The most important mandates, in financial terms, are the requirements that employers provide health services or insurance to their employees, or contribute to social insurance funds for that purpose. Governments can also impose mandates on individuals, as by requiring that children entering school be immunized.
4. Finance health care with public funds. Because mandated insurance is effectively paid for by an earmarked, involuntary contribution which is equivalent to a tax, "public" health expenditure is commonly defined to include such costs along with expenditures from public budgets. The obverse of spending public funds is to tax particular activities or goods, such as alcohol and tobacco, at least partly for health reasons. This issue is not treated here; while taxation which reduces consumption of specific goods may have substantial health effects, it is always limited to very few goods and is not used systematically to promote health. Finally, the state may—
5. Provide or deliver services, using publicly-owned facilities and civil service staff. This is what Ministries of Health in most poor countries do; so do various governmental bodies in many countries at all income levels. Once a society has decided to finance health services with public funds, the choice arises of whether to provide them through public facilities or to pay private producers to provide them. The appropriate way to consider this choice is as a standard "make or buy" decision. The issues for a government are the same as for a private firm, and turn on costs—is it cheaper to produce something than to buy from an outside supplier?— and on the risks and difficulties of enforcing contracts and avoiding fraud when dealing with such suppliers.

Because public financing requires public resources, it is perhaps the crucial choice about state action. However, all the instruments mentioned have costs; even information is not free. The benefits from any intervention have always to be weighed against these costs. In addition, sometimes two instruments overlap, or one requires the use of another:

mandates imply regulation, and public provision usually implies at least partial public finance. And two instruments can be alternatives: for part of the population, governments can either finance health care or mandate financing by employers or other private institutions. Differences in ability to pay make it natural to operate mixed systems of public intervention, such as mandated coverage for the non-poor and public finance for the poor. There are alternatives even within mandated coverage, such as "play or pay" arrangements in which employers can finance health care directly for their employees or pay into a social security scheme.

A CONCEPTUAL BASIS FOR PUBLIC AND PRIVATE ROLES IN HEALTH

The health sector is sufficiently complicated, and the conditions of countries are sufficiently different, that economic theory by itself is an inadequate guide to where the frontier should be drawn between the private economy and state action, or to which state interventions should be undertaken, and in what degree. Non- etheless, theory is essential, particularly where two issues are concerned. Both of these refer to market failure, or circumstances in which private markets either cannot be expected to function at all, or can be expected to yield undesirable outcomes which appropriate public intervention might improve on. Some such failures may occur in any sector of the economy; traditional public finance theory explains these cases and provides guidance for public action. Other possible failures arise where insurance is involved, and for reasons specific to the health sector, present particularly acute problems for health insurance.

Since what the health care sector provides to consumers and beneficiaries are specific activities or interventions, it is useful to organize a conceptual basis according to distinctions among these activities. The next part provides this classification; three subsections elaborate on the peculiarities of each area.

THE THREE DOMAINS OF HEALTH CARE

While the activities that promote, protect or restore health are very heterogeneous, they fall into three natural domains, corresponding to public goods, to low-cost private interventions and to catastrophically costly private goods. These domains are constructed by classifying health-related activities along two dimensions: first by the degree to which they are private or public goods, and second, by how much they cost. Both dimensions refer only to characteristics of particular activities or interventions themselves, not to who consumes them or pays for them. As the descriptions of the three do-mains indicate, private goods are separated into low-cost and high-cost, whereas all public goods constitute one domain, regardless of their cost. The reason for this is that while the costs of public goods matter for deciding whether they should be produced, the issue of market failure related to such goods is independent of costs. With private goods, in contrast, some problems of market failure occur only with those services costly enough to be financed by insurance; and poverty, or the inability to buy even low-cost services, is a distinct reason for public intervention.

This classification of health-related activities does not reserve a place for "merit goods", interventions which everyone "ought to have". To exclude this category is not to deny the social or political importance of views about what people "have a right to". The difficulty is that there is no good way to define such goods a priori, and societies make different choices about them. Moreover, so far as these goods are supposed to justify public intervention, there are often other grounds for state financing, mandating or regulating of the goods or services regarded as meritorious. For example, it is widely believed that all children have a right to immunization, but public promotion of immunization can also be justified by the market failures involved.

A particular intervention occupies a small space in Figure; to indicate how different interventions would be classified into the three domains, some typical health care activities are located approximately. The cost of an intervention can vary depending on many factors, such as how widespread the intervention is; there can also be variation in the public or private good nature of an activity. Because a health system produces a variety of interventions in all three domains, it is spread widely over the space. Figure therefore does not serve to compare different systems.

Public goods are goods or services such that one person's consumption does not reduce the amount available for others to consume. Typically these are goods from which consumers cannot be excluded: if they are made available to anyone, they are available to all, at least locally or temporarily. Since people can consume such goods without having to pay for them, no one will produce them for sale to individual consumers. Therefore they will be produced only if government pays for their production. The notion of a public good is no different in health than in any other sector: wherever such goods or services are to be available, they must be financed by government or some other non- market alternative.

Control of disease vectors and protection of food and water safety are examples of pure public goods in health. Individual action may be ineffective, costly or virtually impossible. Most activities in this category are preventive, but some curative actions are also partly public. And not all preventive interventions are public goods. For example, at low levels of coverage immunization confers some public good benefits—because the immunization of part of the population reduces the likelihood that un-immunized people will become infected—but it still produces mostly private benefit for the immunized individuals.

However, as immunization coverage approaches 100 per cent, the benefit becomes more and more public through the mechanism of "herd immunity": a lone unimmunized individual would be just as well protected as if he had been immunized, and could enjoy this protection without paying for it. When the disease can be eradicated by complete immunization coverage, a pure public good is created. This is an example of how the public or private nature of an intervention may depend on the degree of coverage. When smallpox was endemic, individuals had a strong incentive to be vaccinated, without regard for how many other people were also protected. Now that the disease has been eliminated, everyone benefits.

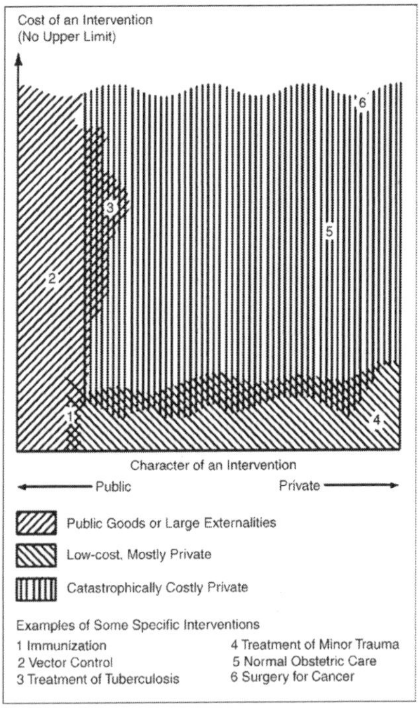

Fig. Three Domains of Health Care

While the distinction between public and private goods is crucial, it does not by itself define the appropriate boundary between private and state action. Moreover, the boundary between public and private goods is not sharply defined, because some interventions provide substantial externalities. In these cases, individuals can and do buy an intervention and benefit from it, but they cannot prevent non-consumers from also deriving some benefit. Because the purchasers do not capture all the benefit, they may be unwilling to pay for all of it: in consequence, private markets can exist but will produce less of these interventions than would be optimal for society as a whole.

This problem arises most readily with communicable diseases, because the infected person puts others at risk. Curing one case therefore also prevents others. Tuberculosis control is a clear example: no victim of tuberculosis is likely to ignore the disease, so there is no problem of people undervaluing the private benefits of treatment. Rather, the cost of treatment—and the fact that they may feel better even though the disease has not been cured—may lead people to abandon treatment prematurely, with bad consequences not only for themselves but for others.

The rest of society therefore has an interest in treating those with tuberculosis, and assuming at least part of the cost. Asymptomatic communicable diseases, such as some sexually transmitted infections, also create externalities; but because people may not realise they are infected, the demand for care is too low even when care is free. There is then an argument not only for subsidizing treatment, but for persuading those infected to seek care. Most health care, however, is a pure private good: Figure reflects this by showing public goods as only a narrow band at the left-hand side, with private goods occupying most of the space. Largely or exclusively private activities include most curative care—especially for non-communicable diseases which pose no threat to others—and all rehabilitative care, and also some preventive or "pre-curative" care. They include home treatment, using health-specific purchased inputs, as well as medical or other professional care.

This area shades into the myriad activities of daily behaviour which also affect health, such as diet, exercise, safety precautions, sexual behaviour, and the use of alcohol, tobacco or drugs. Among these activities, child-rearing is of crucial importance, both for the immediate effect on health—young children are especially vulnerable to infections and accidents—and for the formation of life-long habits. The health effects of these behaviours are usually small on a daily or episodic basis, but can be very large cumulatively.

Figure distinguishes among private interventions according as they are cheap or costly. This is not a sharp boundary, because what is affordable for some people is out of reach for others. And activities which are individually not very expensive may have to be repeated often, creating large cumulative expenditures: renal dialysis and physical therapy are examples. Non-etheless it is crucial to distinguish interventions according to whether they can be paid for out-of-pocket, or financed from accumulated savings, or are so expensive as to represent a catastrophic burden. The cost of medical care is catastrophic if a family or individual can meet it only by selling assets, or taking on debt, to such an extent as to leave it permanently poor. It is initially assumed that no one is too poor to pay for interventions in the "low-cost" domain.

In any health system there is always some private out-of-pocket spending, corresponding to the band along the bottom of Figure. Before the modern understanding of disease and medicine, all health interventions were of this kind, and were paid for by consumers or by charity. Historically, health expenditure began in the lower right corner of the Figure and has expanded into public goods and also into very costly private interventions as knowledge, wealth and institutional capacity have increased. While this pattern is general, countries have followed different paths in the expansion.

Interventions which are needed unpredictably, because disease strikes randomly, and are also too costly for households' ordinary budgets or savings to finance, define the domain of catastrophically expensive care. The only way to deal with the combination of high cost and uncertainty about needs is by risk-sharing, in which people finance health care collectively by contributions which are related to the expected expense in the group but not to any individual's likely consumption of care.

Although the boundaries are blurred, the domain of risk-sharing is conceptually quite distinct from the other two. It normally does not extend into the many routine low-cost, health-related activities, because risk is unimportant there. And explicit insurance—a contract between the consumer who agrees to contribute, and someone else who agrees to pay for specified care—is simply not feasible for public goods. Of course, when the government or a private charity pays for public goods, it assumes the financial risk. This can be thought of as implicit insurance, and in this sense all publicly-financed health care is a form of insurance, even if there is no explicit contract and no payment of individual claims.

Risk-sharing presents the most numerous and complex issues for public policy. The growth in total health care costs is concentrated in this domain because it includes the catastrophically expensive activities. It also shows the greatest variety of institutional arrangements, including substantial participation by private but non-profit providers and financing institutions.

The reason is that while insurance is the natural solution to the risk of needing costly interventions, private insurance markets tend to fail in ways that affect both efficiency and equity, and different institutions represent different partial solutions to those failures. These problems are quite distinct from the inability of markets to deliver public goods or to assure the right level of production of goods with significant externalities.

The question is how and how far governments can and should try to correct for the failings of the insurance market, and whether public finance is necessary or whether other instruments can be substituted for it. Because neither economic theory nor common sense provides as much of an answer as in the domains of public goods and low-cost interventions, judgments in the domain of risk-sharing are more tentative and depend more on empirical information.

Intervention for Public Goods in Health

By definition, public goods cannot be sold in private markets and so create a straightforward justification for collective action. However, the good or service also must be worth the required public expenditure: simply being a public good is an insufficient condition for state intervention. To take an extreme example, erecting giant fans to blow away polluted air would provide a public good, but would almost surely cost too much to be justified. The questions to answer then are, which goods are sufficiently public that private markets cannot provide them adequately? and how should they be valued to determine whether it is justified to pay for them?

As to the first question, governments usually try to provide such indisputably public goods as disease surveillance and sanitary inspection. They often err, however, by trying to cover too wide a range of interventions; Ministries of Health sometimes appear to regard all of health as a public good. An alternative explanation is that they regard all health care as a merit good; the belief that everyone has an unlimited or ill-defined right to free care is sometimes enshrined in legislation or national constitutions.

When public financing is insufficient to fulfill that promise, and particularly when public provision is poorly managed, the result is likely to be both inefficient and inequitable. Governments may err in another way, by recognizing that it can be efficient for the public sector to supply a service—the alternative being to regulate private provision—but subsidize it when most users could pay for it. Water supply and sanitation services are good examples; they generate large public health benefits but are non-etheless mostly private goods for which non-poor consumers are willing to pay.

Still, the state is not always wrong when it treats a largely private good as if it were entirely public. The most striking example is immunization. Had it been left to private markets during the last few decades, it is inconceivable that today some 80 per cent of the world's children would be immunized against the six major vaccine-preventable childhood diseases. Treating the Expanded Programme of Immunization as a public good made possible high coverage even in very poor countries—often higher than in the United States, which has relied more on private finance and provision.

This "mistake" doubtless imposed some costs, in the form of public expenditure which was unnecessary because some people would have paid for immunization privately, and in the distortions caused by the taxes to pay for the programme.

But such costs are negligible in comparison with the health gains. And the public intervention in organizing and largely financing the EPI did not crowd out, but probably stimulated, much private participation in both the financing and the delivery of vaccinations.

The second question is how to value a public-good health intervention. This is the natural domain of cost-effectiveness and cost-benefit analyses. If the only benefit from an intervention is improved health, it does not matter whether that is measured in health terms or monetized. When there are also significant collateral benefits, different approaches can lead to different rankings of interventions.

This is the case for education, water supply and sanitation, and other activities which are valuable for health but also for other reasons—and which may not be justified for the health benefits alone. Cost benefit or cost- effectiveness comparisons are also relevant to public intervention in the other domains of health care, but they are particularly important for public goods for which no private market prices exist.

The issues of which activities to consider public, and whether they deserve to be financed publicly, are difficult. Non-etheless, there are several reasons why this is the simplest domain in which to determine public policy. There is broad agreement on the substantial benefits from a few crucial interventions, which are extremely cost-effective. Individual poverty is not a major source of problems, as it is with private goods: only society's overall capacity to pay matters. Individual ignorance or absence of demand is also of little importance. Finally, this area does not contribute much to the explosion of health care costs, and its financial importance declines as income rises.

The Public Role in Low-cost Private Interventions

This domain includes so many different activities, which are undertaken repeatedly and usually have little health impact per episode, that continued, universal, direct public intervention is simply impossible. Governments cannot be responsible for everyone's daily life, and can probably contribute most by improving households' capacities to look after their own health. Promoting development generally— not only increased incomes but more education and access to all kinds of knowledge, goods and services—seems to be the best way to do this.

How far interference in people's ordinary behaviour is justified, depends on whether the health benefits outweigh the curtailment or modification of individual choices, including non-health benefits. Apart from indefensible extreme positions—for example, that only health matters, and is worth any price; or that only people's private appreciation of their own utility matters, and should be treated as sacrosanct—there is no straightforward answer to this question. Public action cannot be justified simply because of a health improvement; neither can it be rejected just because individual liberty might be limited. Specific public intervention for improved health may be justified under three conditions: ignorance or incomplete knowledge, externalities, and the failure of adults to act as appropriate agents for children.

Each of these involves some kind of market failure, or violation of the private market assumption that rational adults are making informed choices and paying the consequences of their decisions.

The First Problem is Ignorance

People might take better care of their health if they knew how. For example, vitamins are crucial to health but are not observable in food, and people may already believe untruths about diet that help cause vitamin deficiencies. In general, ignorance on the part of one or both parties to a transaction is a major source of failure in the health care market. Of course, "perfect decision making is not ever possible, so the real issue is when the government can or ought to intervene in the information market to improve the market's performance".

Moreover, information is not entirely free, and people do not always act on it. Thus while the cost-effectiveness of efforts to make behaviour more efficient can be very high, it is also quite variable, and people's reactions to information are hard to predict.

Correcting ignorance is not simply a matter of telling people something new, but a larger question of changing beliefs and behaviour. Where better knowledge alone does not lead to changed behaviour, regulation or mandates may also be justified even though they imply more intrusive or coercive intervention. In all such cases, the difficult question is how far it is legitimate to try to change people's views of what they want or what is good for them. Information often complements these other instruments, to reduce opposition to them or improve their effectiveness. The interaction between information and other instruments of behaviour change is seen clearly in the successful effort to reduce smoking in the United States. This situation raises a second problem, of exter-nalities, or interactions among presumably informed adults. Driving while drunk is an example, as is dumping feces or trash in communal water supplies.

These activities impose both health damage and financial costs on others, and individual protection may be impossible or very costly. The chief instrument for public action is regulation, perhaps supported by mandates; these instances do not typically require public finance of health care activities. They may of course also require negative mandates, in the form of laws against certain activities or behaviours.

In practice, there is no sharp boundary between this and the first problem, because some of the behaviour that imposes costs on others may also arise from ignorance: thus reducing the harm from a particular behaviour may require both information and monetary, legal or other incentives. It is more effective to criminalize drunk driving if people are also informed of the dangers, and the health damage can be limited by mandating the use of seat belts.

The third condition is an agent-principal problem and, in contrast to the externalities just discussed, is intergenerational. Children are not yet informed, sovereign adults; they are vulnerable not just to accidents and disease but to the indifference and even sadism of their parents. This problem is somewhat similar to the situation of doctors acting as imperfect agents for their patients.

However, patients often can choose and contract with the doctors who act as their agents, whereas children have no choice of who acts for them. What should the state do when parents are inadequate agents for their children? Requiring that children be immunized is relatively easy, but it is harder to deal with childbeating or exposure of children to secondhand smoke, and still harder to confront parents' beliefs in such matters as sexual education. Where sexual behaviour, vehicle use and consumption of alcohol, tobacco and drugs are concerned, these issues continue through adolescence. This is an exceptionally contentious topic, where it is hard to draw the frontier between public and private responsibilities. Different societies have adopted different solutions, and there is often bitter disagreement within societies over the rights and duties of parents and the degree to which the state can or should interfere in family life.

There are potentially very large health gains at stake in this debate: eight or nine of the ten worldwide leading causes of illness in young children are substantially correctable at low cost and four of these—diarrheal disease plus three nutritional deficiencies—can be largely controlled by the family, with little public expenditure. These diseases account for about 20 per cent of young children's ill health; the total share of child health that depends on parental behaviour is of course substantially larger.

In all these instances, the principal instruments of state action should probably be information and regulation. Mandates are justified for a few activities such as requiring schoolchildren to be immunized, or that foodstuffs be fortified, and against a few other activities. Substantial public finance, however, is usually justified only because some people are too poor to pay for health-related goods and activities, whether these involve medical care or such necessities as food.

Risk-sharing for Catastrophically Costly Private Goods

When risks cannot be fully controlled, and the associated costs may be catastrophic, the only solution is to share the risk. None of the features of this domain is unique to health care, but the magnitude and interaction of certain problems are especially important in health care markets. Moreover, the health risk is only partly associated with income or employment, and the financial risk is hardly associated at all with income or occupation.

Health insurance differs sharply from insurance for non-human assets such as homes or vehicles, where the value of the asset, and therefore the cost of insurance, is usually related to income. Another fundamental difference is that medical care allows for preventive maintenance and for repair, but not for complete replacement of the damaged capital, which in this case is a human body. Insurance for non-human assets operates in just the opposite way, protecting against the loss of the asset but not paying for its upkeep. Insurance may even cover the cost of a temporary substitute for the lost home or vehicle, which is impossible with health insurance. Risks are also harder to estimate for health insurance, both because of the inherently much greater complexity of the body than of non-human property and because there are often different possible treatments for a given health problem, with different costs, outcomes and risks.

Insurance against health risks raises some well-known difficulties leading to various kinds of market failure. One such problem arises because insurance is a contract by which someone other than the patient agrees to pay for his or her health care. As with all contracts, there is an incentive for the insured to behave differently because of the insurance; this is called moral hazard. One consequence is that consumers who do not pay the full cost of health care will consume more of it. This is desirable, since the point of insurance is to let people consume health care they could not otherwise afford. It means, however, that the price must cover the increased demand that results from insurance, and not simply the care that people would otherwise want to buy out-of-pocket.

In theory, there are two potentially more worrisome problems associated with this moral hazard. The first is that people may not only consume more medical care generally, but care that costs too much relative to its effectiveness, yielding smaller health gains per dollar spent. The second risk is that people may take poorer care of their health via daily activities, because they pay the full cost of those, but only part or none of the cost of the resulting increased curative care. Both problems imply excess resources being dedicated to health care.

They may also imply worse health, if increased curative care does not fully compensate for reduced prevention and protection. Some degree of moral hazard is intrinsic to all kinds of insurance, but it is more limited in the case of non-human assets because the insurance does not cover ordinary wear and tear. And cheating the insurer, by burning down one's house or abandoning one's car and reporting it stolen, is illegal, to prevent the insured person from fraudulently collecting cash.

Such compensation is generally not possible under health insurance. Moral hazard in health insurance is independent of how it is financed, so it does not by itself determine whether insurance should be paid for privately or publicly. A consumer who voluntarily buys private insurance ends up paying for the additional medical care consumed by other purchasers, and judges whether this cost is justified by his or her own greater access to care. When insurance is paid for by taxes or mandatory contributions, however, this choice cannot be made.

Moral hazard may then justify controls on what public money is used for, to avoid expenditure on interventions of little health value which consumers would not voluntarily agree to buy for other people. There is scant empirical evidence on the importance of these problems, particularly as to whether insurance leads people to be more careless about their health than they would be if uninsured.

As to the relation between insurance and less cost-effective medical care, the evidence in the United States is that higher out-of-pocket cost for medical care does not make consumers choose more cost-effective services, and may even make poor consumers forego highly justified care. Except in the latter case, there is little evidence that making the consumer pay higher costs under insurance leads to worsened health.

Inefficiency in a competitive insurance market also takes the form of excess purchases of insurance—that is, insurance for interventions which could be more efficiently financed out of pocket or insurance which leads to needless or unjustified use of medical care. This is inefficient to the degree that it leads to excess administrative costs for handling numerous small claims, and because of the excess consumption of health care. Private insurers can only partly control this tendency through deductibles. This problem arises partly because of ignorance: people tend to overestimate small risks and may buy too much insurance even when they pay its full cost. Moral hazard, however, is a greater problem: people who do not pay the full cost of insurance will buy too much of it, just as with medical services.

Market failure in the form of over-insurance happens primarily through the tax system. Many governments allow private employers to treat insurance cost as an expense, but then—in contrast to salaries— do not treat the value of insurance as income to workers. Subsidy through the tax system is notorious in the United States both for insurance for workers which is financed by employers and for part of the Medicare insurance for the elderly. It is estimated that employer-financed insurance would decline by one-sixth or more in the absence of this subsidy, and that in consequence the overall demand for medical services would fall by about five per cent.

Alternatively, governments directly subsidize social security health benefits out of general revenue. General revenues are used to support social security systems throughout Europe and Latin America. In Chile, payroll taxes can also be used to finance private insurance. All these direct and indirect subsidies to insurance are not only inefficient, but highly inequitable when only part of the labour force is covered. The poor typically benefit only when coverage is universal.

When various profit-maximizing insurers compete to sell insurance, there are two further and closely related problems, of adverse selection on the part of consumers and of risk selection on the part of insurers. The former refers to selection of customers which would be adverse to the interests of insurers— fundamentally, it describes the danger of enrolling people who would cost more on average than the insurance could finance. This can happen because the amount of insurance coverage people want and are willing to pay for depends partly on their knowledge of their own health conditions and risks. People who expect to need little health care are unwilling to pay as much as those who expect to need much care, so a policy costly enough to cover high- risk people will lose out in the market to a cheaper policy adequate for low- risk people.

Universal coverage at the same price for everyone may therefore be impossible to achieve, or may not generate enough revenue to finance all the health care demanded. To protect themselves against the combination of low premiums and high potential costs, insurers engage in risk selection or "cream- skimming": they spend more on administration, or create barriers to enrollment, to screen out high-risk individuals or conditions. Such "underwriting", as it is called, is particularly costly for individual applicants for insurance, and gives rise to large scale economies because when a large group is enrolled, the insurer needs to estimate only the average risk of needing care.

This practice is the natural market response to the problem of adverse selection. Inefficiency takes the form of increased administrative costs, and also increased health risks for those excluded from insurance. Particularly when pre-existing conditions are not covered, people with health problems who are insured by their employers cannot readily change jobs without losing their insurance; other differences in insurance coverage may also create "job lock" among workers.

This labour immobility is another source of inefficiency, of unknown magnitude. One answer to the problems of adverse and risk selection is price differentiation according to risk, which is theoretically efficient in that it allows everyone to have the insurance he or she is willing to pay for. Such price variation is common to other forms of insurance: for example, rates for automobile insurance often vary by age and by the way a vehicle is used.

Unfortunately, there are serious difficulties with letting the market create comparable differentials in health insurance. One is that some people are willing to pay only a small amount, because they expect to need little medical care. Faced with a price that would cover the cost of care for everyone, they will not purchase insurance. When they drop out of the market, the price of coverage for those who expect to need more care is driven up because the risk is spread over fewer and higher-cost people.

Even if they are willing to pay more than those who anticipate needing very little care, the price of insurance may rise beyond their capacity to pay. They will be unable to buy insurance, despite a willingness to pay more than the average consumer. Such failures do not occur in other insurance markets because risks are more uniform or predictable, or more closely related to income.

Of course, people's willingness to buy insurance depends on their expectation about future needs for medical care, and they may guess wrong. People who are young and healthy today, and therefore unwilling to spend much on insurance, may when they are older want much more medical care than they now anticipate. But if they become willing to buy substantial coverage only late in life, the cost will be higher than if it were spread over a longer period, so they may be unable to pay for insurance once they recognize the need for it. The difficulty of predicting health care needs is exacerbated by the rapidity of technical change in this sector.

Another problem with differential prices is that despite the importance of many behaviours for specific health problems, rather little of total health risk is under the individual's control. People cannot be held personally responsible for much of their ill health since it is genetic in origin, or due to the actions of others. Often the best that people can do by controlling their own behaviour is to postpone problems, which is very valuable but does not necessarily save money over a lifetime.

Behavioural change may also take a long time to show effect on the burden of disease or the volume of treatment. Because so little health risk is under people's control, behaviour-related prices—whether for health care or for insurance itself—are of only limited value in making markets work.

One can charge people for smoking or for not wearing seat belts, or reward them for careful driving but prices are not feasible for most health-related behaviours. People have some choice of where to live and whether to drive a car, but no choice about inhabiting the body they were born with. Notions of fairness are involved in the choice of how far to allow or control price differentiation in health insurance, because people often do not think others should be punished financially, in addition to their physical suffering, for bad luck. In addition, the possibility of death or substantial permanent disability sometimes makes treatment urgent. Adverse selection is therefore a problem of equity as well as of efficiency.

The problems of moral hazard and adverse selection arise partly from the fact that consumers and insurers possess only incomplete information, which causes market failure in the sense that markets work perfectly only when both buyers and sellers possess full information. Of course, insurance is wanted in the first place because people do not know what will happen to their health, and they agree to share risks when they do not know what will happen to others' health. A further complication is that of information asymmetry: information available to only one side of a market readily leads to market failure.

For example, consumers who know their health risks have an incentive to conceal them from insurers so as to avoid higher premiums. They also know how they have modified their behaviour, or mean to do so, because of insurance. Insurers, in contrast, generally know more than consumers about average risks and about costs of care; consumer ignorance of these matters can also lead to inefficiency.

Unfortunately, it does not follow that the problems of incomplete and asymmetric information could be corrected just by supplying information. Better knowledge on the part of consumers about health risks may lead to more efficient purchase and use of insurance. However, obtaining the information needed to restore symmetry would be impossible or very costly; too much is still unknown about how much people can control their health through behavioural choices. Even if it were symmetrically available to consumers, insurers and providers, more information might make it easier for insurers to practice risk selection and discriminate among customers, and thereby exacerbate inequity. In fact, in an unregulated market, this is the probable consequence of the increasing availability of information linking genetic endowment to the likelihood of developing specific illnesses or health problems.

Information asymmetry also arises between patients and doctors, since the latter typically know much more about medical conditions and treatments. Patients may accept, or even demand, treatments they would not buy if fully informed, but which are advantageous, financially or otherwise, to medical professionals.

There is however little firm evidence as to how much of this potential "supplier-induced demand" actually occurs. In any case, this is not simply a problem of rich countries, where most people have insurance and therefore do not worry about costs; it has also been documented in poor societies where lack of education and information may make it particularly easy to exploit consumers.

In summary, the consequence of these market failures is that in an unregulated, competitive private market in third-party insurance those with chronic conditions or high health risks will be under-insured, administrative costs will be higher than necessary because of insurers' efforts to screen out risks and the costs of processing claims in a market with many insurers and many providers, and procedures of low or questionable value will be performed because neither the provider nor the consumer pays for them. It is in these specific senses that "the market does not work" in health care; these are primarily failures of the insurance market rather than shortcomings of the market for health care itself.

Private markets have developed other forms of insurance which reduce, but do not eliminate, these problems, such as health maintenance organizations. Under this arrangement, providers also act as insurers and assume the risk. Insofar as this controls costs by shifting the burden to suppliers of medical care rather than to consumers or third-party insurers, it may allow more coverage of the chronically ill, and may reduce the utilization of relatively ineffective procedures. However, without some form of public intervention such arrangements will have little effect on the problems caused by poverty and adverse selection. The question remains which kinds and degrees of public intervention can best mitigate the problems inherent to private insurance markets without introducing worse inefficiencies or inequities.

MARKET FAILURE AND HEALTH CARE NEEDS

Since the unregulated, unsubsidized private market is the extreme alternative to government intervention in health care, much of the debate as to appropriate public and private roles in the sector turns on whether, how, and how badly markets may fail. Market failure, as an economic notion, refers to possible mismatches or disequilibria between what the market supplies, and what fully-informed, rational consumers of health care would demand. It does not deal with the concept of need for health care, which is theoretically an unsatisfactory concept but is also difficult to do without.

People want health care not for any intrinsic utility but because they think they need it, that if care is not provided their health will deteriorate or fail to improve. In contrast, much of the criticism by both health care professionals and consumers of how health systems operate deals explicitly with needs. Just as demand and supply may be out of balance, there can be imbalance between demand and need or between need and supply of services. Market failures in the narrow economic sense are among the reasons for these imbalances.

Some failures result from barriers to the operation of competitive private markets in bringing supply and demand together. Others distort demand from what it would be if based on complete and symmetric information and if there were no public goods or externalities; this causes imbalance between demands and needs. While competitive private markets are generally the best way to bring demand and supply together, they are much worse suited to make either demand or supply match people's needs. Public intervention in the health market, in contrast, is aimed at satisfying those needs, and runs the corresponding risk of failing to take account of demand.

Either a purely private or a purely public health care system is likely to control one of the three potential imbalances, at the cost of failing to control or even worsening one or both of the others. This is a major reason why most health care systems are far from being all private or all public.

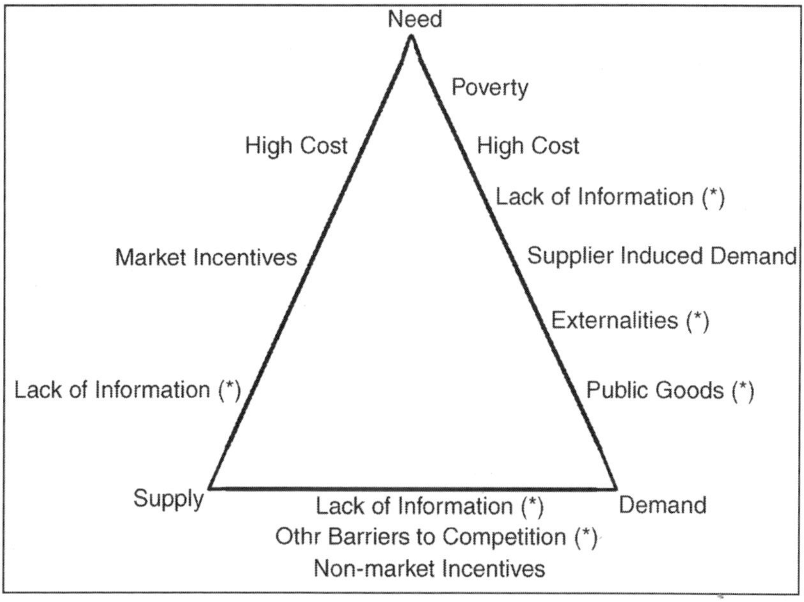

Fig. Need, Demand and Supply for Health Care

DEALING WITH POVERTY

In the discussion thus far, it has been assumed that no one is too poor to buy a variety of health interventions out of pocket. Similarly, it is assumed that no one is too poor to buy insurance against catastrophic health risks; people differ in income and in their assessment of risks, but everyone can afford some insurance.

A Minimal State Role in the Absence of Poverty

Under these conditions the state's role in the domain of private, inexpensive health-related activities would be limited mostly to information and regulation; there would be no reason to finance this kind of health care publicly if everyone could afford it out-of-pocket. In the domain of risk-sharing, people who chose not to buy insurance, or bought too little of it, would have to pay for care out of pocket or do without it. Because doing without care would sometimes pose the risk of avoidable death, some kinds of care— emergency services, at least—are typically available even to the uninsured. People's willingness to let others suffer the consequences of imprudence does not usually include letting them die because they bought too little catastrophic protection.

This kind of imprudence constitutes moral hazard, and unlike some behaviour on the part of insured people, it cannot be dealt with by differential premiums. Motorcyclists who prefer not to wear helmets can in principle be charged more for their insurance, just as smokers can; the more difficult problem is how much care to provide for the uninsured cyclist whose injuries are worse because of failure to wear a helmet.

This situation provides a justification for enough public finance or mandated insurance to cover the cost of a few crucial services to which everyone would have access and for which everyone would have to pay through taxes.

If there were no poverty, then, the role of the state in the health sector might be relatively limited, and would—except for the minimum insurance requirement just described—concentrate on the adequate provision of public goods and the correction of market failure in the domain of risk-sharing. Whether in order to correct or compensate for that failure the state should mandate or finance insurance beyond that minimum of emergency care, is a question of the social efficiency of doing so, rather than leaving insurance to the private market.

The fact that insurance would not need to be subsidized—the removal of an equity justification for interfering in the insurance market—does not mean that governments should do nothing, because the efficiency failings of private voluntary insurance are as important as the inequities to which it gives rise.

How Poverty Complicates Public Roles

The existence of poverty, of people too poor to buy many "inexpensive" health activities or an "adequate" amount of insurance, complicates the question of what the state should and should not do in several ways. These complications are not limited to the domains of private goods, because problems of public health are often more severe among the poor. They are likely to be at particular risk from contaminated air and water and so to benefit more than the non-poor from public health interventions and they often suffer more serious consequences from common illnesses. In general, imbalance between need and demand may be more important where the poor are concerned, because they have less knowledge on which to base their wants for health care as well as less resources with which to express demand.

Medical indigence is in most respects no different from poverty with respect to food and other basic needs, and, as with those needs, the rest of society may agree to subsidize the poor. The difference is that poverty relative to predictable, low-cost needs such as food can be dealt with either by transfers or subsidies in kind, or by supplementing income. With health, the risk of needing very costly care generally makes it more efficient to deal with medical indigence by subsidizing insurance than through income transfers. However, there is little experience in most poor countries in subsidizing private providers or insurers to meet the health needs of the poor.

This requires government administrative capacity and appropriate pricing mechanisms, to prevent excess provision and even outright fraud, which has been a major problem, for example, in Brazil.

A public subsidy to private insurance, as an alternative to dealing directly with large numbers of providers, also requires premiums differentiated by age, sex or other conditions, to reduce the scope for risk selection and make it feasible to mandate universal coverage. In consequence, one of the most important effects of poverty is that it makes public provision, with all its typical problems, look attractive or even necessary in poor countries.

Aside from the problems of regulation, it is financially difficult to provide the poor with the same level of services enjoyed by those already covered by private or social insurance. Even extending social security coverage to the poor, to replace the more limited services offered by Ministries of Health, would be very costly in many Latin American countries.

Public provision often means poor health care for the poor, but public financing of private services would not easily solve the underlying financial problem even if it led to improved quality of care. Finally, in countries where all public money now flows through government or parastatal facilities, shifting to public finance of private providers requires that public hospitals and clinics be privatized or at least given sufficient autonomy and capacity to manage themselves and compete for public funds against other providers. Such changes are potentially very valuable, but they are likely to be particularly difficult, since public facilities need to be exposed to some financial risk without the danger of collapse in publicly funded provision.

The difficulty of incorporating the poor into the same insurance schemes which cover the non-poor, whether by extending social security coverage or by subsidizing the purchase of private insurance, leads to efforts to create insurance specifically for the poor, typically at the community level.

Any such scheme is intrinsically limited by the low incomes of participants, so it cannot finance very costly interventions and can only yield subsidies from the less poor to the more poor. It may non-etheless be appropriate when the insurance is meant to pay for only such health care as can also be provided locally and which therefore is not very costly—although perhaps still catastrophic for a poor family to finance.

Unfortunately, the problems of moral hazard and adverse selection arise even in these circumstances. For example, if insurance is sold for short periods to accommodate families' fluctuations in income, then, as occurred in Burundi, people may buy the "health cards" entitling them to services only when they are already sick or can anticipate a medical need. That effectively eliminates the difference between an insurance payment and a fee, and reduces the amount of money that can be raised by the scheme.

These problems lead to complications such as rewarding people who use less health care by reducing the cost of their cards for the next period or by charging an additional fee or "fine" to those who pay for insurance only when ill. Such incentives work against moral hazard and adverse selection, but if they are large enough to have much effect they may greatly reduce the scheme's revenue or the demand for services. And administrative expenses may absorb a large share of revenue.

Poverty also creates or strengthens reasons for the state to intervene in low-cost, health-related activities, whether these are inexpensive medications and services or such non-medical items as food supplements. Some interventions can be accommodated by broadening public health services, for example by including micronutrient supplements or treatment for intestinal parasites.

Others can be covered by financing private providers, such as the clinics which operate under "covenants" with the Brazilian social security system. However these activities are dealt with, poverty pushes governments to finance a wider range of low-cost interventions and to rely less on information and regulation. If this were the only force at work, it would lead to a larger public share of health expenditure in poor than in rich countries, simply because there are more poor people who cannot pay for those interventions.

In the sum of health spending, however, this effect is overwhelmed by the tendency of governments to mandate or finance more insurance for the non-poor, as income rises.

A third effect of poverty is to limit the use of prices to curtail demand or control costs. Being poor already greatly constrains demand, and poor people are necessarily more sensitive to prices for health care than the non-poor. This means both that user fees can raise relatively little revenue from the poor, and that unless there are offsetting improvements in quality, utilization may be sharply reduced. The experience with user fees has been extensively analysed, notably in Sub- Saharan Africa in connection with the Bamako Initiative.

There is evidence that—as might be expected—utilization declines, sometimes sharply, if fees are raised but nothing else changes. There is rather less information on service characteristics, such as whether user fees improve the availability of drugs. And almost nothing is known about the impact on health outcomes or on system efficiency or cost-effectiveness.

Fees are sometimes set arbitrarily or with inconsistent criteria; charges low enough to have no effect on the poor may or may not be worth collecting; and targeting by exempting the destitute from fees does not have to be expensive but there is a risk of high administrative costs and low net revenues. The same problems arise for collecting insurance deductibles and co-payments from the poor.

Not only does poverty increase the risk of ill health; sickness and disability can make or keep people poor. The relation between health and poverty is sometimes regarded as another reason for the state to invest in health, in order to raise productivity. However, the fact that some health care increases incomes is not a separate objective for government action. If health care made people so much more productive that the extra income could pay for the health care, then in perfect markets people could borrow against their future productivity. When capital market failures prevent such borrowing, and those failures cannot be corrected directly, then any public intervention—such as financing the health care or providing loans to consumers—that secures the health gains will also yield the increase in productivity.

JUSTIFICATIONS AND RISKS OF STATE INTERVENTION

As the foregoing analysis shows, there are three distinct, independent arguments for governments to intervene in health care rather than leaving it entirely to private markets. One is to ensure the optimal level of production and consumption of public goods and goods which have a partly public character because of externalities. These can be health care services themselves, activities protective of health, or information that helps people take better care of their health and make better use of services.

A second reason is to make insurance work more efficiently and more equitably, for those services which can be produced in private markets but for which risk- sharing is required because of high costs and uncertainty about needs. The third reason is to subsidize those too poor to buy insurance or even, sometimes, those inexpensive activities and services which the non-poor can afford out of pocket. These three reasons derive from the three domains of health care defined by cost and by the public or private nature of services. Market failures underlie two of these reasons, but in different ways. In the case of public goods and externalities, the failure arises from the nature of the good or service. In contrast, problems in insurance markets arise from the way the good is financed. None of the three reasons is unique to the health sector, but all are more important in this sector than in much of the rest of the economy.

The arguments for not leaving health care and health insurance to uncontrolled private markets are all arguments that efficiency or equity can be improved, if the state intervenes appropriately. They are not arguments that anything the public sector does, will improve matters. Just as there is a well-defined set of market failures typical of the health sector, there are consistent government failures, ways in which governments act to create worse outcomes than could be reached, and in some respects even worse outcomes than markets would generate.

The most common and severe criticism of public action concerns provision: especially in poor countries, governments offer medical care which is supposed to be free to users, on equity grounds, but which is centrally-controlled, under- financed and of poor quality in both medical and human terms. Because the budgets of public facilities often are unrelated to service output, and civil service rules make it difficult to fire, transfer or discipline unproductive staff, the costs of health gains may be very high even if salaries and other input costs are low.

And the pervasive lack of incentives for efficiency means that capital is also bought in excess, not maintained, and under-utilized. The result is that even rather poor people, the supposed beneficiaries of the public system, often pay out of pocket for those private services they can afford. This makes them pay twice for some of their care, exacerbating the inequities arising from the tax system and from difficulties of access due to the geographic location of facilities.

Governments typically fail where provision is concerned, by trying to do too much and by competing with private providers only in price terms— that is, subsidizing provision rather than competing on quality and satisfaction. With respect to the other instruments of state action, failures are more varied, and often result from doing too little rather than too much.

This is likely to be the case particularly for regulation and for the dissemination of information. Mandates show a very mixed pattern: middle- income countries in particular often mandate insurance for part of the population through social security schemes, but do not effectively mandate either insurance or care for everyone. Richer countries, in contrast, appear much less prone to government failure largely because they rely much more heavily on regulation and mandates, and much less on public provision. Where public facilities are important, as in some European countries, they operate under greater autonomy than in poor countries, and this is balanced by greater regulation of private providers. The result is to concentrate more on the right roles for public action, and less on dividing the health sector into disjointed private and public spheres. The distinction is particularly important because in many countries, the two sectors overlap greatly: the same professionals work part-time in each, private providers often use public facilities to treat private patients, and so on.

To provide public goods and to subsidize health-related activities for the poor, two of the three main reasons for state action, both require public finance. In both these areas there is also room for the other instruments of state action; and the problems associated with risk sharing can lead to various combinations of interventions, which may or may not include spending public money. Societies therefore have much latitude in how much, and by what means, the government intervenes in health care markets, just as they have in deciding how much to spend on health in relation to income and to their health problems or needs.

THE APPROPRIATE PUBLIC ROLE IN HEALTH

As a first approximation, it is easier to say what govern-ments should not do in health than to specify what they should do. That is, it is clear that certain actions are likely or certain to violate one or more of the objectives of a health care system to an important degree. To apply a topographic metaphor: such actions correspond to falling off a plateau of satisfactory outcomes, all somewhat different but none clearly dominating the rest, and into one of the surrounding chasms of one or another kind of failure. Four "don'ts" are discussed in what follows: they refer to the way the public is taxed, charged or exempted to pay for health care; the providers to which governments transfer public funds; the way providers are paid; and the services they are paid to provide.

WHAT GOVERNMENT SHOULD NOT DO

The first thing governments should not do is to use the tax system, or any system of fees at public facilities, to make the poor subsidize the health care of the rich. Conceptually, subsidies are justified only for the poor, and broader financing of care through insurance is a question of efficiency rather than of equity.

This is not only a matter of whether the rich use more of publicly-financed services than the poor do, although great inequities often arise because the rich have more access to those services. Financial equity also depends on who pays the taxes. More narrowly, governments should not contribute to social security financing from general revenues, unless coverage is universal, because when only part of the population is covered it is usually the poor who are excluded. And governments should not treat private insurance coverage as a cost to employers unless it is also treated as income to beneficiaries. Such practices are not only inequitable; they are also inefficient to the extent that they lead to excessive spending on health care, or reduce labour mobility. Controlling inequitable subsidies does not mean that social security systems should be dismantled or must be made universal. Even when incomplete, such mandated insurance includes substantial progressive subsidies from high- paid to low-paid workers, and the mere fact that some people in society receive more generous health care is not necessarily a problem, so long as they pay for it. What matters is that governments not make everyone pay for what some are excluded ex ante from receiving. Perverse subsidies not only cause immediate inefficiencies or inequities, they also create interests that oppose subsequent health system reform.

This is evident in the United States and Chile and it is the reason why the design of subsidies is a crucial part of any reform to extend or improve coverage for the poor. The second thing governments should not do is tie public finance to public provision. The choice of whether to provide care through public or parastatal facilities should be treated as a "make or buy" decision, subordinate to the larger decision about what to pay for. That does not necessarily mean eliminating public provision, which will sometimes be the best solution. It means rather that competition between public and private providers should be based on costs and on quality, and not on price to the consumer, as is commonly the case.

To achieve those goals, however, requires other changes in how public institutions operate, changes that probably cannot occur so long as public funds go automatically and exclusively to government facilities. This conclusion is most pertinent to poor countries where public systems are most likely to be inefficient and to be used only because they are free or nearly so. High-income countries with a large share of public provision, particularly in hospitals, suffer less from these problems.

A third thing governments should not do is pay for health care by fee-for- service, unless other mechanisms are used to control expenditures. This is seldom a problem with publicly provided services, but makes it hard to control costs when governments finance private providers. Even negotiating or controlling the fees is not enough, as the Canadian experience demonstrates, since providers can respond to fees they consider too low, by increasing output. This helps explain why Canadian health expenditure has risen faster than that in European countries which rely on other payment mechanisms.

European countries which pay for health care by fee-for-service also rely on global budgets, utilization reviews or other instruments of cost containment. Since expenditures equal prices times quantities, and since quantities of services respond to prices and are difficult to control directly, countries which pursue both macroeconomic and microeconomic efficiency in health spending usually control both prices and expenditures. In contrast to European and North American experience, Brazil applies this system to block grants for federal expenditure in states with relative financial autonomy; but in states where federal money is paid directly to providers, the federal government also controls one crucial quantity, the number of hospitalizations that federal money will pay for. In all cases, the government sets prices for services.

It also helps, in controlling expenditures, to define "services" as complete treatments for specific conditions rather than as all the individual components of such treatments, so they can be financed by mechanisms such as the Diagnostic Related Group payments used in the United States and the provider can be required to assume part of the financial risk. Changing from a system based on overall budgets and on salaries for providers, to a fee-for-service system without offsetting the resulting incentives to overprovision can lead to an explosion of costs, as in the Czech Republic. Finally, if governments mean to pursue some combination of better health and lower costs, they should not—in fact they cannot—simply finance whatever people demand when care is free to consumers.

This does not mean governments should not "subsidize demand" rather than "subsidizing supply" or providing services. It means only that there must be limitations on what will be paid for publicly. Such limitations are a particularly contentious matter, because both good health and cost containment may be opposed to consumer or provider satisfaction, which are also politically important objectives.

Non-etheless, two empirical observations are germane to this decision. One is that private insurance always carries some limitations, either as to the services covered or as to cost-sharing. Except where poverty is important, so that cost- sharing is more difficult, there is no reason for public finance to be systematically more generous in this regard than private risk-sharing arrangements.

The second observation is that private markets will tend to supply what people demand, and public intervention typically acts to emphasize needs instead. In other forms of public subsidy, it is common to distinguish between wants and needs, and concentrate spending on the latter. This is the case, for example, with food subsidies, which are also very much healthrelated. Price subsidies are usually limited to "basic" foodstuffs, and food stamps cannot legally be used to buy alcohol or other non-necessities.

This may be considered partly a matter of efficiency, assuring more health gain than would otherwise occur. But it is also a matter of equity: in contrast to actuarial private insurance, where every purchaser buys the expected value of the health services needed, public finance is involuntary. It comes from taxpayers who have a legitimate interest in meeting needs, and thereby getting value for their money, but not necessarily in paying for wants.

None of these "don'ts" is easy to implement, because some consumer or provider interests can be expected to oppose every one of them, in every country. But they are arguably the most important conclusions about where the public/private frontier should run in the health sector. It is notable that none of these conclusions depends solely on features unique to the health sector.

The peculiarities of health matter most for the difficulty of distinguishing "needs" from wants, and—partly as a consequence—for the dangers of paying providers for whatever they choose to provide, without incentives to control costs. A system which avoided the problems would still present complex and difficult questions for the proper role of the state, but it would have more latitude to pursue improvements. And it would not matter so much, exactly what objectives the government pursued or which combination of instruments it applied.

WHAT GOVERNMENT SHOULD DO

Beyond the prescriptions for how the state should deal with the problems of each of the three domains of health care, several "dos" appear to be generally valid for governments. If the objective is to minimize deadweight losses from public intervention and leave as much room as possible for private choices, then the first thing governments should do is to use each less-intrusive instrument to the point where a more intrusive intervention is justified, following the sequence of increasingly greater interference— inform, regulate, mandate, finance and provide services. That is, governments should regulate private activity when merely improving people's information is not enough, deliver services if it is infeasible to finance private providers equitably, and so on. Public finance is inescapable for some actions, but particularly in low- and middle- income countries much can probably be accomplished by better use of information and regulation. Failure to use these other instruments well, can increase the need for public finance.

Sometimes the problem is that governments exploit these instruments too little. They do not regulate private insurance when it first begins to expand, which makes subsequent regulation politically more difficult; or they do not initially react when health-damaging behaviours such as smoking become more entrenched. Sometimes the problem is inappropriate regulation, which needlessly restricts competition, or enforces inefficiency in the public sector by centralizing nearly all decisions. And poor countries in particular often get the worst of both worlds by paying for activities which should be, but are not, regulated: government subsidy of medical education without adequate control of quality or relation to needs is a common example.

In the worst of cases, governments use all the available instruments in exactly the reverse order. They try to provide more health care than they can pay for, with the result that most services are under-financed and of poor quality; they try to finance services, some of which might be mandated and paid for by consumers or employers; they mandate care, as by social security systems, without adequately regulating it; and they do too little to inform the public and providers either of dangers to health or of how the health care system is actually working.

Much of the criticism of government failure in the health sector, especially in poor countries, describes the result of getting things backwards. These ideas are represented in Figure, which shows the appropriate relation among the instruments by which the state can intervene in health care which portrays the kind of inappropriate or imbalanced relation often found in poor nations. Figure indicates that whatever is mandated, financed or provided publicly should also be regulated, and much else besides. The state can finance some care that is not anyone's mandated responsibility, and can also mandate care or insurance coverage which is financed privately. And most if not all public provision should be fully financed by government, but possibly with much more scope for finance than for provision by the state.

The largest sphere pertains to information, covering activities in which there is no other public interference with the market. In contrast, Figure shows a much smaller effort to inform or regulate, very little use of mandates that are not also publicly financed, and a sphere of provision as large as, or even larger than, that of finance.

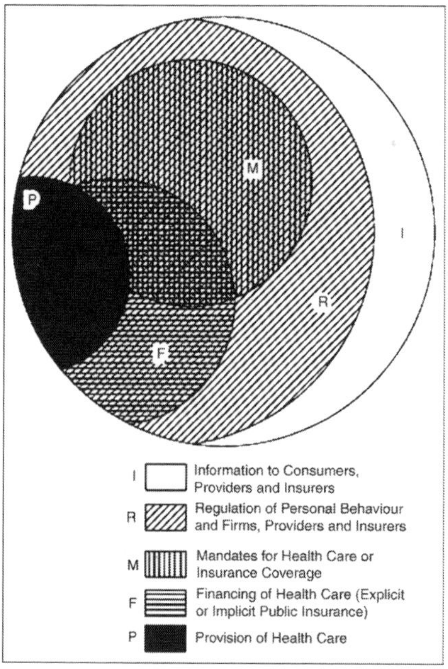

Fig. Appropriate Use of the Instruments of Public Intervention in Health Care

Of all the instruments of public action, regulation may be the most under- utilized. Brazil and Chile both provide examples of the resulting problems. In Brazil, the state finances three-quarters of medical care but directly provides only about one-quarter of it, so the instruments of finance and provision are used in the appropriate order. But there is very little regulation of the competence of medical professionals, of the quality of care, or of the rapidly- growing private insurance industry. The lack of regulation even interferes with financing the system, since private insurers sometimes send their customers to publicly financed facilities without paying for care, and until recently fraud was widespread.

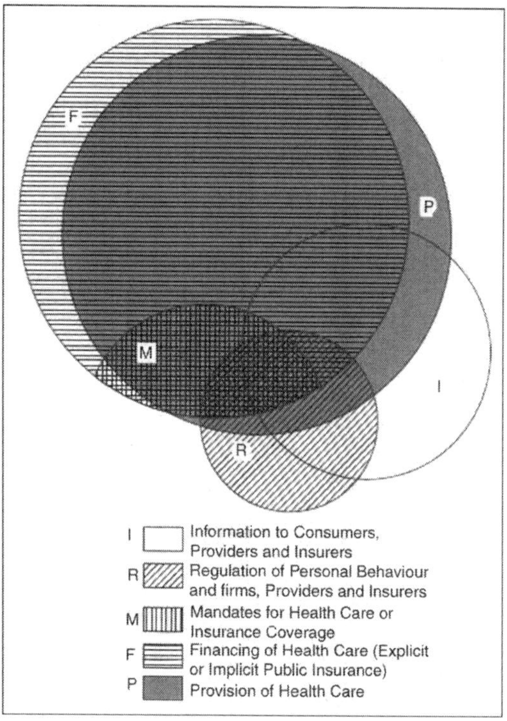

Fig. Typically Inappropriate Use of the Instruments of Public Intervention in Health Care

In Chile, the private insurance industry was created by public action, with essentially no regulation—but with a mandate allowing people to spend on private insurance, the tax contributions that formerly were used to finance the public system. The lack of regulation may not have affected medical quality, but it has worsened the financial situation of public facilities, raised administrative costs, and promoted risk selection. Even more serious failures to regulate have arisen in Eastern and Central Europe, as former state monopolies of health finance and provision have given way to competitive private provision.

A second thing governments should do is to stimulate competition in the provision of health care. This is largely a matter of promoting public/private competition but it also includes removing any unjustified barriers to competition within the private sector, and between for-profit and non-profit providers such as non-governmental organizations. The lack of competition is usually less of a problem in the domain of low cost, health-related activities than in the domain of costlier activities requiring insurance.

This recommendation extends a fortiori to non-medical components of health care such as the "hotel" services of hospitals. How far competition should be carried is not always obvious. For example, whether public facilities should make their own purchasing decisions for such inputs as drugs, depends on whether central bulk purchasing reduces costs while maintaining adequate supplies. Even in the latter case, there should of course be competition among suppliers for such purchases.

As income increases and poverty declines, of course, it becomes easier to pass the burden of cost containment to consumers. However, it does not become medically any more effective or economically any more efficient to do so. Moreover, as income increases the capacity for supply-side responses by providers also increases, so it continues to be preferable to keep cost control incentives on the supply side of the market.

Finally, it is urgent to deal with the pervasive problem of government failure, and to improve the capacity to do whatever government ends up doing. This is especially important when market failures are so important that for the public sector to withdraw, on the ground that it also is subject to failure, would only make matters worse. Much of the criticism that governments, particularly in poor countries, try to do too much in health arises because of how badly they appear to operate, more than from any evidence that they have exceeded some optimum degree of state intervention. More skill and understanding, and fewer internal barriers to efficiency, make sense whether the state's role shrinks, as by leaving more provision to the private sector, or expands, to finance more coverage for the poor. One of the things governments generally need to do better, particularly in poor countries where much private medical practice may be of low quality, is to use regulation, mandates, training and other interventions to help the private sector function better.

This is increasingly recognized as an essential component of almost any health sector reform, and the need for it will only increase as health systems become more expensive and complex. All five instruments of intervention— information, regulation, mandates, finance and provision— need to be used well, and using less of one instrument and more of another will not, in general, reduce the need for governments to perform capably.

❐

Index

❑❑❑